This book is due for return on or before the last date shown below.

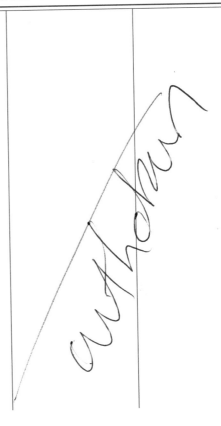

Urological Oncology:
A day-to-day guide
for the non-specialist

Hospital Medicine monograph

edited by Hitendra RH Patel

Quay Books
MA Healthcare Limited

Quay Books Division, MA Healthcare Limited, Jesses Farm, Snow Hill, Dinton,
Wiltshire SP3 5HN

British Library Cataloguing-in-Publication Data
A catalogue record is available for this book

© MA Healthcare Limited 2004
ISBN 1 85642 245 3

Printed in the UK by Cromwell Press, Trowbridge

Contents

List of contributors

Mr Manit Arya, MBChB, FRCS, is Clinical Research Fellow in Uro-oncology, Department of Cellular Pathology, Institute of Urology and Nephrology, University College London, London W1W 7EY

Mr Ahsan Haq, MBBS, MA, MSc(Urol), FRCS(Urol), is Specialist Senior Registrar in Urology, Department of Urology, The Ipswich Hospital, Health Road, Ipswich, Suffolk IP4 5PD

Professor Jean Joseph MD, Section of Laparoscipic and Minimally Invasive Surgery, Department of Urology, University of Rochester, Medical Centre, 601 Elmond Avenue, Box 656, Rochester, NY 14642–8656, USA

Mr Frank Lee, MA, FRCS(Urol), is Research Fellow in Urology, Institute of Urology and Nephrology, University College London, London W1W 7EY

Mr Shikohe Masood, MBBS, FRCS, is Staff Grade in Urology, Medway Maritime Hospital, Gillingham ME7 5NY

Mr Hitendra RH Patel, BMScHons, MBChB, MRCS, PhD, FRCS(Urol), is Honorary Clinical Lecturer in Urology, Institute of Urology and Nephrology, University College London, London W1W 7EY

Dr Venita Patel, MBBS, DRCOG, MRCP(UK), is Specialist Registrar in Paediatrics, Department of Paediatrics, Guys and St Thomas' Hospital, London and Mary Sheridan Centre for Child Health, 5 Dugard Way, off Renfrew Road, Kennington, London SE11 4TH

Mr Iqbal Shergill, BScHons, MRCS, is Clinical Research Fellow in Uro-oncology, Department of Cellular Pathology, Institute of Urology and Nephrology, University College London, London W1W 7EY

Mr Hassan Wazait, FRCS, is Clinical Research Fellow in Uro-oncology, Department of Urology and Minimally Invasive Surgery, Whittington Hospital, London N9

Dedication

To Jai Maadi for inspiration, and my daughter Maanya Devi

Foreword

In the world of cancer, information concerning diagnosis and treatment is rapidly expanding. Keeping abreast of these changes can be a thankless task. The idea for this book came from many different people asking the same questions. While researching each topic, it became clear to me that a book summarizing and distilling the available knowledge would be pertinent. Moreover, simplifying the increasingly long-winded information would allow non-specialists to assimilate quickly the necessary knowledge.

The advent of rapid-access cancer care and cancer networks means that non-specialists' understanding of the basics will help to make the patient journey more satisfying, and decrease the pressures on the National Health Service (NHS). Also, students learning about the subject of uro-oncology will instantly be able to access the knowledge necessary for undergraduate examinations.

Finally, I hope readers, whether lay or professional, will feel that their journey from basic science to the new horizons of uro-oncology have been satisfactorily covered without being overburdened with the minutiae.

Hitendra RH Patel
BMScHons, MBChB, PhD, FRCS(Urol)
Hon Clinical Lecturer in Urology
University College London
November 2003

1

The basic science of uro-oncology

Iqbal Shergill, Manit Arya and Hitendra RH Patel

The progression of a tumour from normal cells to pre-cancerous ones, to cancer and then on to local invasion and finally metastasis is the result of the clonal expansion of cells that have acquired a selective growth advantage, enabling them to outnumber neighbouring cells. The extent of local, regional and distant spread of a cancer must be accurately determined, as this indicates the prognosis and also helps to determine treatment. This chapter outlines the aetiology and pathology of cancer, its molecular diagnosis and the treatment options available.

Introduction

A neoplasm literally means 'new growth', and is the name given to a group of cells that fail to respond to the normal regulatory pathways of the human body. As a result, a neoplasm proliferates in an atypical and uncontrolled manner, with no useful function, and develops into either a benign or malignant tumour; *Table 1.1* highlights the differences between benign and malignant neoplasms. The following discussion concentrates on malignant tumours, as most urological cancers are malignant.

Aetiology and pathology of cancer

The functional state of a cell can be described in terms of the cell cycle (*Figure 1.1*).

The aetiology of cancer is not known, and therefore most cases described are referred to as sporadic. However, certain risk factors have an association with carcinogenesis. For example, environmental factors such as cigarette smoking and exposure to aromatic amines, in rubber and dyes, have a strong correlation with the development of bladder cancer. In addition, ionising and ultraviolet radiation may predispose to cancer. Viral infections such as the human papilloma virus have been implicated in genital cancer, and in 10% of prostate cancer there is a positive family history of the virus (Walsh *et al*, 2002).

The common finding in cancers from all these aetiological groups is that there are accumulated genetic changes, which underlie the development of cancer (*Figure 1.2*).

Table 1.1: Differences between benign and malignant neoplasms	
Benign	Well circumscribed and often encapsulated
	Effects by pressure
	Remains localized
	Rate of growth is usually slow
Malignant	Irregular, ill-defined and not encapsulated
	Effects by invasion and destroying structures
	May metastasize via lymphatics, blood vessels and tissues
	Rate of growth is fast

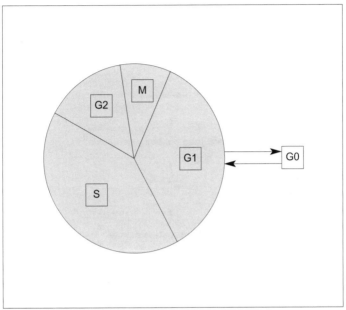

Figure 1.1: The cell cycle. G1 is the phase in which protein and RNA synthesis occurs in preparation for the S phase (DNA synthesis). During G2, protein synthesis occurs prior to mitosis in the M phase, in which the cell finally divides. Throughout this cell cycle, checkpoints exist that maintain the integrity of DNA replication. G0 is the phase in which a cell is quiescent. It is, however, able to be removed from this phase and into the cell cycle, and thus divide by the action of mitogens, nutrients and growth factors. Successful completion of the cell cycle and subsequent cell division results in proliferation and growth. At the same time, some cells undergo cell death, which may be programmed (apoptosis) or caused by abnormalities during the cell cycle. It is the fine balance between the cell proliferation rate and the cell death rate that dictates overall growth of tissues. Essentially, a cancer can be thought of as an abnormality of normal growth, but with the distinction that this growth is abnormal, uncontrolled and with no useful function.

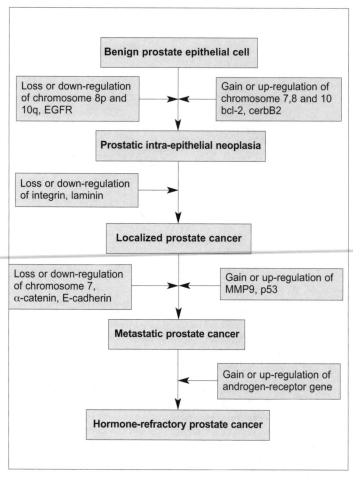

Figure 1.2: Genetic changes in prostate cancer progression. EGFR=epidermal growth factor receptor; MMP9=matrix metalloproteinase 9.

The progression of a tumour from normal cells to pre-cancerous ones, to cancer and then on to local invasion and finally metastasis is the result of the clonal expansion of cells that have acquired a selective growth advantage, enabling them to outnumber neighbouring cells. This may occur by one or a combination of the following ways:

- over-expression or activation of proto-oncogenes (e.g. bcl-2)
- inactivation of tumour-suppressor genes (eg. p53)
- mutations in mismatch repair genes (mismatch repair genes mutL homologue 1 (MLH1) and mutS homologue 2 (MSH2)).

Although a normal cell is thought to require five or more mutations to become cancerous (Nowell, 1976), the probability of this happening is increased because the genetic material in pre-cancerous and cancer cells is intrinsically unstable, a characteristic known as genetic instability.

Proto-oncogenes are normal genes that serve to regulate normal growth. However, the aetiological factors outlined above, and other reasons that are as yet unclear, cause the proto-oncogenes to be converted into oncogenes. The normal function of these genes is thought to be altered by point mutation, amplification or dysregulation, resulting in uncontrolled cell division or invasive growth.

Oncogenes are referred to as dominant genes, as only one copy of the gene requires an abnormality to result in an alteration in function. Conversely, tumour-suppressor genes exert a negative influence on cell growth and therefore inhibit cellular proliferation. Therefore, mutation of these genes results in failure to suppress normal growth restraints.

Tumour-suppressor genes are non-dominant in that both copies of the tumour-suppressor gene need to be abnormal for an abnormal outcome. Knudson's two-hit hypothesis (1971) refers to tumour-suppressor genes specifically described in retinoblastoma.

Two groups of patients were studied who had developed retinoblastoma: young patients with bilateral disease, and older people with unilateral tumours. In the first group it was found that one retinoblastoma gene was mutated at birth and the other was normal. As the retinoblastoma gene is a tumour-suppressor gene, both copies require to be damaged before any abnormality is apparent. The normal gene is mutated early on, as these patients are at high risk of developing a mutation of the single gene. The second group have both genes that are normal. They therefore require 'two hits' to result in an abnormality. As this may take a significant time to occur, the patients are generally in an older age group. Mismatch repair genes simply are present normally to fix genetic damage when it occurs. Damage to these genes is one mechanism that may lead to carcinogenesis.

Malignant tumours are fatal because of their ability to grow into adjacent tissues by invasion, and then spread to a remote or secondary site within the body. This phenomenon is termed metastasis. Initially, as a tumour enlarges >1 mm it requires an independent blood supply to maintain its growth. It does this by producing angiogenic factors that produce areas of vascularization, which subsequently develop into new blood vessels.

To spread to a new location, the tumour cells must increase their motility and detach themselves from the main tumour bulk. To prepare for invasion there is a loss, or down-regulation, of adhesion molecules, which make cells adhere to each other. The classic example of this is E-cadherin; reduced levels of E-cadherin are associated with poor differentiation and increased grade of tumour. Subsequent passage through basement membranes is helped by the presence of proteinases, such as matrix metalloproteinases, with activity against the extracellular matrix. This enables tumour cells to invade into blood vessels. Subsequently, transport in the vascular space occurs until the tumour cells reach their target organs.

Single cells can be killed by the body's own immune system. However, clumps of tumour cells have the ability to survive and get stuck in capillary beds where adherence and extravasation may occur with the help of cell surface adhesion molecules; the end result is a secondary tumour. Survival of secondary tumours then depends on developing a new blood supply aided by the presence of growth factors.

Molecular diagnosis of cancer

It is essential to determine accurately the extent of local, regional and distant spread of a cancer, as this indicates the prognosis and also helps to determine treatment. Currently, assessment is based on the histopathological study of both cells found at the margins of tissue removed during surgical resection of cancer, and of cells found while draining lymph nodes of the cancerous area. The problem with this approach is that small foci of metastatic cancer can be missed, either because the sampling is insufficient or because the analysis of the cell morphology is uninformative.

The ability to use molecular markers to detect a small number of cancer cells in pathological specimens should improve clinical staging. Because molecular genetic changes in general are responsible for the biological characteristics of neoplastic cells, it is likely that specific genetic alterations will predict the behaviour of such cells. It is hoped that the time will come when oncologists will be able to characterize the molecular fingerprint of a tumour, which represents the genetic profile of a tumour. Such a fingerprint might then provide clues to help to determine whether a tumour will be fast- or slow-growing, whether it will metastasize, and whether it will respond to particular treatment regimens.

Although the molecular fingerprinting of tumours is not yet a clinical reality, the value of molecular markers in clinical practice has already been suggested by many research studies of the clinical implications of various genetic markers for different types of tumours (van de Vijver *et al*, 2002). The genetic profile of a tumour, its molecular fingerprint, will improve the ability to predict tumour behaviour, and thus help to determine optimum treatment. In addition, specific genetic changes can be predictive of tumour behaviour (eg. response to treatment); they can, therefore, define prognosis and might help to optimize treatment. Also, screening of asymptomatic patients will be possible with genetic methodology.

The possibility of identifying neoplastic cells in clinical samples using molecular genetic techniques was first demonstrated in 1991, when Sidransky *et al* detected cells in urine samples from patients with bladder cancer that had mutations of the p53 tumour-suppressor gene, which were identical to the mutations found in the cells of the primary tumour. Subsequently, it has been shown that a p53 mutation could be detected in a urine sample nine years before the diagnosis of bladder cancer was made (Kirk, 1999).

In clinical practice, the usefulness of particular molecular methods depends upon several factors, including the:

- sensitivity of clinical tests
- specificity of clinical tests
- positive–predictive value of clinical tests
- feasibility and cost of carrying out clinical tests in large numbers
- acceptability of the clinical test to patients.

Sensitivity of clinical tests

The sensitivity of a clinical test for cancer is defined as the proportion of the total number of patients with cancer tested that were correctly identified by the test. For molecular genetic assays, this depends on the:

- proportion of cancer cells in which the abnormality is found
- ability of the test to detect abnormal cells in a clinical sample.

We know that mutations, deletions, translocations and duplications of many genes can contribute to tumour formation, depending on the tissue of origin; however, no single genetic change is common to all cancers, a fact that will limit the sensitivity of any test to detect a cancer.

The successful detection of abnormal cells in clinical specimens requires the use of methods that selectively enrich for specific mutations. Thus, genetic detection is currently limited to the study of point mutations at a few known, fixed sites. Microsatellite instability might prove to be a more useful screening test for some tumours; for example, microsatellite analysis has been found to have a sensitivity of 95% in detecting bladder cancers that had been confirmed by cystoscopy, compared with only a 50% sensitivity for conventional cytology (Mao *et al*, 1996).

Specificity of clinical tests

The specificity of a clinical test for cancer is defined as the proportion of the total number of people tested that were correctly identified by the test as not having cancer. Because some specific genetic abnormalities are thought to be a characteristic of cancer cells, some molecular genetic tests should be highly specific. However, other genetic abnormalities can also be characteristic of dysplastic and pre-cancerous cells; thus, until more is known about the natural history of such lesions (for example, the proportion of lesions that progresses to invasive cancer, and over what time scale), the specificity of such markers to cancer is hard to predict.

The positive–predictive value of clinical tests

The positive–predictive value of a clinical test is defined as the proportion of the total number of people tested who test positive and who really have the disease. Thus, it is a function of both the sensitivity and specificity of the test and of the prevalence of the 'condition' in the population that is being screened. Because the prevalence of cancer in screened populations is usually low, sensitivity and specificity must be high if the positive–predictive value of a cancer screening test is to be acceptable for clinical use.

Feasibility and cost of carrying out clinical tests in large numbers

Clearly, a molecular test has to be cheap and easy to perform in all clinical settings for it to be acceptable. Currently no such molecular test is available, but work is in progress to develop such an assay.

Acceptability of the clinical test to patients

Ideally a non-invasive test (voided urine) or a minimally invasive investigation (blood test) would be the ideal test for molecular investigation. Consenting patients to more invasive procedures (biopsy) makes the test much less acceptable. In addition, with such an emotive diagnosis such as cancer, patients require a test to ideally have a 100% sensitivity and specificity.

Treatment options

Chemotherapy

Chemotherapy is the use of cytotoxic agents to destroy malignant disease while sparing surrounding normal tissues. The treatment is based upon the cell cycle of malignant and normal cells, and outcome depends on the rate of growth of tumours. In the majority of urological cases, the main use of chemotherapy is in the management of metastatic disease, and therefore treatment is systemic in nature. A notable exception to this generalization is the use of local intravesical treatment of some bladder tumours.

Chemotherapeutic agents act on different stages of the cell cycle and are preferentially toxic to malignant cells as compared with normal cells. This principle is based on the observation that the rate of proliferation of cancer cells is greater than that of normal cells, and they are therefore more susceptible to genetic damage from chemotherapeutic agents. Indeed, tumours that are rapidly growing, such as germ cell tumours, are more chemosensitive than slow-growing tumours, such as prostate and kidney tumours. In addition, tumours have a high growth rate early on in their lifetime, which then slows down as the tumour bulk enlarges. As such, chemotherapy will be less effective in larger tumours.

Pharmacokinetics reveal two classes of chemotherapeutic drugs — those that are phase dependent, and those that are phase independent.

Phase-dependent chemotherapeutic drugs. These can only kill cells during G2 of the cell cycle. They are effective at low doses, but have the disadvantage that higher doses will not improve their efficacy in cancer cell death; examples include etoposide, methotrexate and vinca alkaloids (*Table 1.2*).

Phase-independent chemotherapeutic drugs. These result in exponential cell death according to dose, and are equally effective in causing cell death in the cell cycle as well as in G0, the resting phase; examples include alkylating agents, actinomycin, 5-fluorouracil and anthracyclines (*Table 1.2*). As their mode of action is to kill cells in the cycle, invariably some normal cells will also be affected. The main toxicity is therefore to normal cells that have the highest rates of cell-cycle turnover. These include bone marrow, gastrointestinal mucosa and hair, resulting typically in cytopenia, mucositis and alopecia, respectively. In addition, nephrotoxicity, neurotoxicity, haemorrhagic cystitis, pulmonary fibrosis and cardiotoxicity are less common complications.

Systemic therapy administered after a patient has been treated with another modality is termed adjuvant therapy. Patients at low risk of relapse following curative treatment should not undergo adjuvant treatment as they are at a higher risk of getting toxicity than any benefit of survival. This depends on an assessment of the risk of relapse. Proposed adjuvant therapy must be shown to reduce the risk of relapse and increase the rate of disease-free survival in a phase-III trial (Bolla *et al*, 1997, 2002). Finally, as this group of patients are generally cured and therefore asymptomatic, toxicity must be kept to a minimum. Treatment should be administered before any surgical resection. Advantages include early treatment of potential micrometastases and debulking of large tumours to allow complete resection. Again, there must be good evidence from phase-III trials to show clinical benefit of disease-free survival with a reduced risk of relapse. Indeed, there are few indications for this in urological oncology. One example are patients with germ cell tumours of the testes and known metastatic disease.

Table 1.2: Mode of action of different chemotherapeutic drug groups, with examples of drugs available

Alkylating agents	Produce their effects by linking an alkyl group (R-CH-) covalently to chemical moeities in protein and nucleic acids • Cyclophosphamide • Cisplatin
Antimetabolites	Structurally homologous to normal substrates interfering with cell mechanics • Methotrexate • 5-Fluorouracil
Anti-tumour antibodies	Bind to DNA and between base pairs • Doxorubicin • Bleomycin
Plant-derived agents	Bind to tubulin, affecting protein synthesis in microtubules • Vinca alkaloids • Etoposide
Antibiotics	Interpose between DNA strands, interfering with template function • Actinomycin • Anthracyclins
Biological agents	Anti-tumour effects by modulating normal defence mechansism • Bacille Calmette-Guérin (BCG)

Specific problems of treating urological malignancy with chemotherapeutic agents also includes renal insufficiency from obstructive uropathy caused by the disease, with the nephrotoxic actions of many of the drugs making things worse. In addition, dose adjustments need to be made in patients with ileal conduits and reabsorption problems, as well as dealing with lowered bone marrow reserve in patients with pelvic disease and previous radiotherapy.

Radiotherapy

Radiotherapy has been used to treat genitourinary malignancies for more than a century, with reports of radiotherapy treating prostate cancer in the early 1900s (Walsh *et al*, 2002). Radiotherapy uses the principles of ionising radiation to treat malignant tumours. Radiotherapy treatment requires the treatment of the primary tumour, a margin of 0.5–1 cm surrounding it for micrometastatic spread and a further 0.5 cm to accommodate for technical reasons. A large field of radiation is therefore required.

During treatment, radiation is commonly produced by machines such as the linear accelerator (X-rays), but may also be produced by radioisotopes, in the form of beta particles or gamma rays. Biologically, these forms of radiation are indistinguishable. An X-ray consists of photons (high-energy pockets), which interact with molecules of body tissues, resulting in ionization and release of electrons. These electrons cause direct damage to DNA, or if generated in the presence of oxygen have an indirect action by forming peroxide radicals, which result in damage to double-stranded DNA. In both cases, the effects of radiation damage occur only when an affected cell undergoes mitosis; cells may still be able to continue to maintain their normal physiological functions.

Normal cells are able to respond to radiotherapy damage in a more favourable manner than tumour cells, by higher rates of repopulation than tumour cells, thus conferring an advantage. In addition, there is evidence that DNA damage causes programmed cell death or apoptosis, especially in germ cell tumours of the testes. Fully differentiated tissues that are incapable of dividing or where the cell cycle is extremely long, such as in the heart, muscle and spinal cord, may never express the effects of radiation, or do so at a much later stage than active cells, such as those found in the bladder and urethra.

Instead of giving a whole dose of radiation in one visit, the total dose is divided into small parts over a period of time. This is called fractionation, which has the following benefits. Reducing the dose per fraction enables normal tissues to repair DNA damage more effectively than tumours. Many tumours contain hypoxic areas, and most radiotherapy treatment is oxygen dependent; as the tumours become smaller, the hypoxic areas are exposed to oxygen enabling further treatment with radiotherapy to be more effective.

The effects of radiotherapy also depend on the size of tumour, histological subtype and tolerance of normal tissues. Whereas most tumours of the bladder, prostate and urethra may be treated with cumulative doses of 65 Gray, comprising single, daily doses of 1.8–2.0 Gray, larger tumours may require up to 80 Gray of total dose radiation. In addition, renal cell carcinoma is relatively resistant to the effects of radiotherapy, whereas squamous transitional cells and adenocarcinomas and seminomas are sensitive. Indeed, some tumours may be so sensitive that they require even less dose than is standard. Seminomas are such an example, requiring around 25 Gray for satisfactory treatment.

The complications of radiotherapy are summarized in *Table 1.3,* but are dependent on the total dose of radiation administered, the dose per fraction and the volume of normal tissue irradiated.

Brachytherapy

Brachytherapy is a relatively new form of therapy, where radioactive sources can be placed in close proximity to (interstitial brachytherapy), or sometimes within (intracavity brachytherapy) a tumour. Interstitial therapy involves needles, catheters or seeds in tumours of the prostate, bladder, penis or periurethral tissues; intracavity brachytherapy involves inserting the radioactivity into an orifice, such as in penile or urethral cancer. The advantages are that high doses over a relatively short period of time can be delivered without the side effects of conventional treatment. The main disadvantage is that it is a highly specialized form of treatment limited to a few centres in the country.

Other new forms of therapy include cryotherapy, laser and high-intensity focused ultrasound.

Table 1.3: Complications of radiotherapy	
Acute complications	Skin inflammation
	Mucositis and oesophagitis
	Bone marrow stem-cell suppression
Chronic complications	Stem-cell effects
	Connective tissue damage
	Vascular damage
	Lymphatic obstruction
	Second malignancy in future, such as ovarian, endometrial and bladder

Conclusions

In this chapter the core and basic concepts underlying oncology have been introduced, the aetiology and pathology of cancer have been discussed and the molecular diagnosis and treatment options for this disease have been contemplated. The aim has been to develop a background knowledge of oncology, to enable an understanding of the various urological cancers discussed in this book.

References

Bolla M, Gonzalez D, Warde P *et al* (1997) Improved survival in patients with locally advanced prostate cancer treated with radiotherapy and goserelin. *N Engl J Med* **337**(5): 295–300

Bolla M, Collette L, Blank L *et al* (2002) Long-term results with immediate androgen suppression and external irradiation in patients with locally advanced prostate cancer (an EORTC study): a phase-III randomised trial. *Lancet* **360**(9327): 103–6

Kirk D, ed (1999) *International Handbook of Prostate Cancer*. Euromed Communication Ltd, Haslemere

Knudson AG (1971) Mutation and cancer: statistical study of retinoblastoma. *Proc Natl Acad Sci USA* **68**(4): 820–3

Mao L, Schoenberg MP, Scicchitano M *et al* (1996) Molecular detection of primary bladder cancer by microsatellite analysis. *Science* **271**: 659–62

Nowell PC (1976) The clonal evolution of tumour cell populations. *Science* **194**: 23–8

Sidransky D, Von Eschenbach A, Tsai YC *et al* (1991) Identification of p53 gene mutations in bladder cancers and urine samples. *Science* **252**: 706–9

van de Vijver MJ, He YD, van't Veer LJ *et al* (2002) A gene-expression signature as a predictor of survival in breast cancer. *N Engl J Med* **347**(25): 1999–2009

Walsh PC, Retik AB, Vaughan ED, Wein AJ, eds (2002) *Campbell's Urology*. 8th edn. WB Saunders, Philadelphia

Key points

- A neoplasm literally means 'new growth', and is the name given to a group of cells that fail to respond to the normal regulatory pathways of the human body. As a result, a neoplasm proliferates in an atypical and uncontrolled manner, with no useful function, and develops into either a benign or malignant tumour.

- Although a normal cell is thought to require five or more mutations to become cancerous, the probability of this happening is increased because the genetic material in pre-cancerous and cancer cells is intrinsically unstable, a characteristic known as genetic instability.

- Oncogenes are referred to as dominant genes, as only one copy of the gene requires an abnormality to result in an alteration in function. Conversely, tumour-suppressor genes exert a negative influence on cell growth and therefore inhibit cellular proliferation. Therefore, mutation of these genes results in failure to suppress normal growth restraints.

- Chemotherapy is the use of cytotoxic agents to destroy malignant disease while sparing surrounding normal tissues.

- Radiotherapy uses the principles of ionising radiation to treat malignant tumours.

- Brachytherapy is a relatively new form of therapy, where radioactive sources can be placed in close proximity to (interstitial brachytherapy), or sometimes within (intracavity brachytherapy) a tumour.

2

Prostate cancer: management and controversies

Jean Joseph and Hitendra RH Patel

Advances in the management of prostate cancer are associated with uncertainties and controversies in screening, who and when to treat, the best treatment option for localized disease and what to do with biochemical relapse after presumed curative treatment.

Introduction

Prostate cancer is now the most common cancer diagnosed, and the second most common cause of cancer death in men (Lee *et al*, 2002). Improvements in the detection of prostate cancer include prostate-specific antigen (PSA) testing and transrectal ultrasound-guided biopsy of the prostate. These enable the detection of the disease at an early stage when it is organ-confined and amenable to curative treatment. Refinements in surgical and radiotherapy techniques provide the opportunity to maintain the patient's quality of life by reducing the risk of complications. However, there are still unanswered questions, such as the efficacy of population screening, the treatment modality that gives the best survival and quality of life in localized disease, the management of biochemical relapse and the pathology of hormone-refractory cancer.

Epidemiology

There has been an increase in the incidence of prostate cancer and in the resulting mortality. By 1990, prostate cancer had become the second most common cause of death in men in England and Wales (Majeed and Burgess, 1994). The incidence of prostate cancer in the UK in 1996 was 21 400, and the number of deaths from prostate cancer in 1998 was 9460 (National Statistics Office, 2002).

Aetiology

Prostate cancer has no known aetiology. It is classed as a sporadic cancer; however, men are at a higher risk if their immediate relatives have prostate cancer.

The relevant causal gene for familial prostate cancer is found on chromosome 1 (Carter *et al*, 1993). The factors implicated for developing prostate cancer are shown in *Table 2.1*. John *et al* (1995) found no conclusive evidence that vasectomy was a risk factor.

Pathology

Prostate cancer is a multifocal and heterogeneous disease. Most prostate cancers are adenocarcinomas that arise from high-grade prostatic intra-epithelial neoplasia (Burton *et al*, 2000). This is present in 4.0–16.5% of needle biopsies and is strongly predictive of co-existing carcinoma, thus warranting a repeat biopsy (Wiley *et al*, 1997). Many interesting and unusual morphological variants of prostate cancer have been identified, but they account for <10% of cases. However, these variants need to be recognized and differentiated from benign variants, and it must be known that their clinical behaviour may differ from the usual prostate adenocarcinoma.

Table 2.1: Risk factors implicated in the development of prostate cancer		
Factor		**Risk**
Age		Advanced age
Ethnic origin		AfroCaribbean origin
Positive family history		Early age (<55 years)
Diet	Fructose	Low
	Selenium	Low
	Vitamins D and E	Low
	Phyto-oestrogens	Low
	Lycopene	Low
	Fat	High

Grading

The Gleason system (Gleason, 1992) is the most widely used grading system for prostate cancer. It gives a grade (1–5) to the most and the second-most dominant architectural pattern of differentiation. The grade increases as the degree of differentiation decreases. If the most dominant pattern is graded 5 and the second most dominant pattern graded 4, this is described as a Gleason grade of 5+4, or a Gleason score of 9.

Staging

A commonly used system of staging prostate cancer is the TNM (tumour, node, metastasis) classification (*Table 2.2*). Clinical staging is the assessment of the extent of the tumour using digital rectal examination (DRE), PSA and imaging modalities, such as transrectal ultrasound, computed tomography, magnetic resonance imaging or bone scan. Determination of the local extent of the tumour by DRE is referred to as T-staging.

Pathological staging is more useful than clinical staging as a prognostic indicator because only the former can provide data on tumour volume, surgical margin status, extent of extracapsular spread and the involvement of the seminal vesicle(s) and pelvic lymph node(s). However, this information can only be obtained from radical prostatectomy specimen and not radiotherapy (no specimen). Therefore, accurate comparison between surgical and non-surgical treatment modalities continues to be limited.

Diagnosis of prostate cancer

The diagnosis of prostate cancer is made from history, examination and investigations (*Figure 2.1*). Early, organ-confined prostate cancer can be asymptomatic as the majority (70%) arise from the peripheral zone of the gland, away from the urethra. As the tumour grows, symptoms can develop as a result of local and/or metastatic effects (*Table 2.3*). In men presenting with lower urinary tract symptoms, it is important to exclude prostate cancer if the diagnosis and treatment would have a significant impact on the patient's survival.

Table 2.2: The TNM staging system for prostate cancer

TNM	Description		
TX	Primary tumour cannot be assessed		
T0	No evidence of primary tumour		
T1	Clinically inapparent tumour, not palpable or visible by imaging	T1a	Incidental tumour found at transurethral resection of the prostate in which ≤5% of the resected tissue is cancerous
		T1b	As in T1a, but >5% of the resected tissue is cancerous
		T1c	Cancer detected by needle biopsy of the prostate
T2	Palpable tumour confined to the prostate	T2a	Tumour involves one lobe
		T2b	Tumour involves both lobes
T3	Tumour beyond capsule (locally advanced)	T3a	Extracapsular extension
		T3b	Seminal vesicle involvement
T4	Tumour is fixed or is invading surrounding structures other than the seminal vesicles	T4a	Tumour invades bladder neck and/or external sphincter and/or rectum
		T4b	Tumour invades levator muscles and/or fixed to pelvic wall
NX	Regional lymph nodes cannot be assessed		
N0	No regional lymph node involvement		
N1	Metastasis in a single regional lymph node, maximum ≤2 cm		
N2	Metastasis in a single regional lymph node, maximum diameter between 2–5 cm; or multiple lymph node metastases, none >5 cm maximum diameter		
N3	Metastasis in a regional lymph node >5 cm in diameter		
MX	Presence of distant metastasis cannot be assessed		
M0	No distant metastasis		
M1	Distant metastasis	M1a	Involvement of non-regional lymph nodes
		M1b	Involvement of bone(s)
		M1c	Involvement of other distant sites

TNM=tumour, node, metastasis

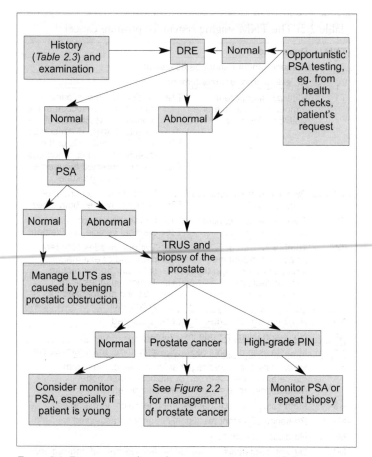

Figure 2.1: Diagnostic pathway for patients presenting with lower urinary tract symptoms or suspected prostate cancer. DRE=digital rectal examination; LUTS=lower urinary tract symptoms; PIN=prostatic intraepithelial neoplasia; PSA=prostate-specific antigen; TRUS= transrectal ultrasound.

Table 2.3: Effects and symptoms of prostate cancer

Effects	Symptoms
Local effects (from growth of prostate cancer into neighbouring structures, eg. prostatic urethra, ejaculatory ducts, neurovascular bundle innervating the corpora cavernosa, distal ureter)	Obstructive voiding symptoms, eg. hesitancy, variable flow, terminal dribbling
	Irritative storage symptoms, eg. urgency, frequency, nocturia, urge incontinence
	Haematospermia
	Decreased ejaculate volume
	Erectile dysfunction
	Symptoms of renal failure
Metastatic effect (from involvement of bone, pelvic lymphatic or venous drainage)	Bone pain
	Anaemia
	Lower limb oedema

DRE

DRE is the primary method for assessing the prostate. However, it is examiner-dependent and has inter-examiner variability (Smith and Catalona, 1995). Many early prostate cancers will be missed by DRE alone (Brawer *et al*, 1992).

PSA testing

PSA testing has revolutionized the diagnosis, staging and management of prostate cancer. PSA is a serine protease produced almost exclusively by the prostatic epithelium and peri-urethral gland in men. Although low concentrations of PSA are produced by the endometrium, breast tissue, adrenal and renal carcinoma, it is sufficiently organ-specific in clinical practice.

However, PSA is not specific for prostate cancer because it can also be raised by manipulation (transrectal ultrasound, biopsy, cystoscopy), in urinary retention, in prostatitis and in benign prostatic hyperplasia. The latter can cause diagnostic dilemmas if the PSA is mildly elevated (4–10 ng/ml), as this can be the result of either benign prostatic hyperplasia and/or cancer.

To improve PSA sensitivity and specificity, PSA density, PSA velocity, age-related PSA and the free/total PSA ratio have been used. All increase the accuracy of diagnosing cancer, but the last method appears to be the most promising (van der Cruijsen-Koeter *et al*, 2001).

Transrectal ultrasound and needle biopsy of the prostate

Although transrectal ultrasound can detect prostate cancer as a hypoechoic lesion, benign processes such as prostatitis or infarction can have a similar appearance; furthermore, not all prostate cancer is hypoechoic on ultrasound. The use of colour Doppler ultrasonography to detect the hypervascularity of cancer may improve sensitivity.

Nevertheless, transrectal ultrasound is essential in performing a systematic needle biopsy of the prostate (Littrup and Bailey, 2000). Complications of needle biopsy include haematospermia (45.5%), haematuria (23.6%) and low-grade fever (4.2%). With the use of prophylactic antibiotics, the risk of developing septicaemia and prostatitis is <1% (Rietbergen *et al*, 1997).

Guidelines

Guidelines by the British Association of Urological Surgeons suggest that PSA testing and needle biopsy should only be performed after the proper counselling of suitable patients. These tests should not be used on inappropriate patients, such as in the elderly or in those whose co-existing medical morbidity has already severely compromised life expectancy (Dearnaley et al, 1999). *Table 2.4* shows the chance of detecting cancer on prostatic biopsy after DRE and PSA results are known.

If cancer is detected, the overall chance of organ confinement can be calculated using Partin's tables (using initial PSA, clinical staging and biopsy Gleason scores; Partin *et al*, 2001). Clinicians have been using these figures to counsel patients when deciding upon curative treatment, such as radical prostatectomy.

Table 2.4: The possibilities of detecting prostate cancer on needle biopsy of the prostate after DRE and PSA testing

DRE	PSA (ng/ml)	Chance of cancer on needle biopsy (%)
Normal	<4	6
Normal	>4	23
Abnormal	<4	15
Abnormal	>4	56

DRE=digital rectal examination; PSA=prostate-specific antigen

Treatment of prostate cancer

Early (localized) prostate cancer

Figure 2.2 gives a management pathway for early prostate cancer. This is organ-confined, and if treated appropriately offers the best chance of cure. There are three treatment options:

• watchful waiting
• radical radiotherapy
• radical prostatectomy.

Watchful waiting is usually offered to men with low-grade, low-volume disease (<0.5 ml), who have a life expectancy of <10 years. Radical radiotherapy can be offered to any group of patients, but is more appropriate for surgically high-risk men. This can be delivered via external beam (conformal) irradiation or implantation of radioactive seeds (brachytherapy). It is usually combined with cyto-reductive hormonal therapy (neoadjuvant and/or adjuvant androgen suppression). Radical prostatectomy is the preferred option for younger and fitter men, with the intention of curing an organ-confined disease on clinical staging. However, up to half of these men have extracapsular disease on pathological staging, preventing a curative operation.

The selection of treatment option is not evidence-based, but is derived from informed choices made by patients and their relatives, with assistance from the clinician. Fully informed patients are made aware of the potential complications from radical prostatectomy and radiotherapy (*Table 2.5*), as well as the side-effects of medical therapy (*Table 2.6*). Lu-Yao and Yao (1997) found the difference in disease-free survival of patients with localized disease between these three treatment options was 10–20%; however, patients with poorly differentiated tumours had a higher ten-year disease-specific survival rate after radical prostatectomy (Gerber *et al*, 1996).

Locally advanced prostate cancer

Although radical prostatectomy (*Figure 2.2*) is often inappropriate because of the unacceptably high local and distant recurrence rate, some urological surgeons consider this option in a few selected patients. Radical radiotherapy (with cytoreductive hormonal therapy) is unlikely to be curative, but will delay local progression. The remaining patients in this group who do not have radical treatment will receive androgen suppression with or without maximal androgen blockade.

Maximal androgen blockade. This involves suppressing testosterone production from the testes (by orchidectomy or luteinizing hormone-releasing hormone agonists) and adrenals (by antiandrogens), which in turn inhibits the stimulation of prostatic cells (cancerous and benign). The theory is attractive and resulted in years of conflicting reports on its efficacy, including the statistical validity of the studies involved. A meta-analysis showed a modest 2–3% improvement in five-year survival using maximal androgen blockade compared with castration (medical or surgical) alone (Prostate Cancer Trialists Collaborative Group, 2000).

Table 2.5: Common potential complications after radical prostatectomy and radiotherapy

Complication	Radical prostatectomy	Radical radiotherapy
Erectile dysfunction	Yes	Yes, less common in radiotherapy
Urinary incontinence	Yes	Yes, less common in radiotherapy
Anastomotic stricture/ bladder neck stenosis	Yes	Yes
Bladder irritation	Yes, usually transient	Yes
Rectal irritation	No	Yes

Metastatic prostate cancer

The main treatment for metastatic prostate cancer is androgen suppression (*Figure 2.3*); about 70% of patients respond to this treatment. Apart from bilateral orchidectomy, a number of agents are available (*Table 2.6*). Unfortunately, almost all of these patients will relapse after a period and develop hormone-refractory disease (*Figure 2.2*). There is no consensus in the management of this difficult situation. When this happens in patients who are on maximal androgen blockade, it is worth stopping the antiandrogen as up to 50% of patients show a drop in their PSA, albeit transient. Second-line hormonal therapy entails a cocktail — steroid plus stilboestrol (after breast-bud irradiation) plus aspirin or warfarin (to reduce thromboembolic events).

Table 2.6: Common side-effects of medical treatment for advanced prostate cancer

Agent	Side effects
Luteinizing hormone-receptor agonists	Hot flushes
	Erectile dysfunction
	Decreased libido
	Osteopenia
	Anaemia
Non-steroidal antiandrogens	Gynaecomastia
	Diarrhoea
Cyproterone acetate	Fluid retention
	Erectile dysfunction
	Hepatic dysfunction (rare but widely known)
Stilboestrol	Gynaecomastia
	Erectile dysfunction
	Cardiovascular toxicity including thromboembolism

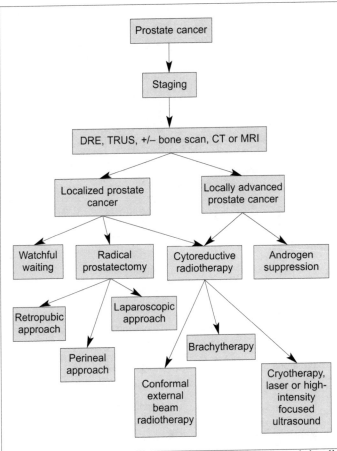

Figure 2.2: Management pathway for early (localized) and locally advanced prostate cancer. CT=computed tomography; DRE=digital rectal examination; MRI=magnetic resonance imaging; TRUS=transrectal ultrasound.

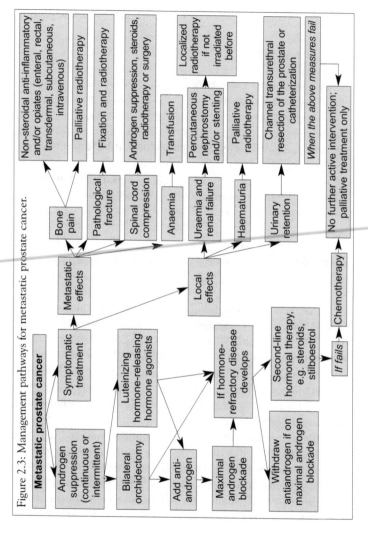

Figure 2.3: Management pathways for metastatic prostate cancer.

Chemotherapy has been tried, although the results with single agents, such as estramustine or vinblastine, have been relatively disappointing. However, the early results using taxanes, such as paclitaxel, in combination with other agents, such as estramustine, were promising (Murphy, 1999), with half of the patients showing a drop in PSA.

The prognosis is poor if patients do not respond to second-line treatment. Renal failure can be caused by the encroaching prostate cancer undermining the distal ureter. The priority is to decide with the patient and relatives whether to proceed with active intervention (percutaneous nephrostomy with or without antegrade stenting) or palliative management.

Screening

Early detection and aggressive treatment is the only chance to cure prostate cancer. PSA-based screening advances the diagnosis by six to ten years and results in a significant stage reduction. However, the patient's survival benefit and the effect on the patient's quality of life from population screening are at present unknown. There is also concern about over-diagnosis, and current UK practice has recommended that its role must be subjected to valid controlled trials before instigation.

Controversially, the American Cancer Society and the American Urological Association have ignored the fact that no valid trial exists to show that screening for prostate cancer reduces prostate cancer-related deaths; they have instigated guidelines to offer all men ≥50 years and men ≥45 years in high-risk groups an annual PSA and DRE (Smith *et al*, 2001).

On the horizon

Apart from research on therapeutic agents to improve the prognosis of advanced prostate cancer (*Table 2.7*), there are controlled trials investigating the benefits of screening and the

Table 2.7: Agents being studied for the treatment of prostate cancer

Agent	Example
LHRH receptor antagonist	Abarelix
17,20 lyase inhibitors (MAB in a single agent)	Abiraterone acetate
Endothelin receptor antagonist	ABT-627
Angiogenesis inhibitor	Angiostatin
	Thalidomide
Cell-cycle inhibitors	DNA synthesis inhibitor suramin
Combined (type 1 and 2) 5-alpha-reductase inhibitor	Thymidine kinase ganciclovir adenovirus
	Cytosine deaminase gene product
Adnovirus/suicide gene therapy	
Immunotherapy	Granulocyte-monocyte-colony stimulating factor vaccine
	Allovax
	Dendritic cells to present PSA to T cells
Apoptosis agonists	Anti-sense Bcl-2 oligonucleotides

LHRH=luteinizing hormone-releasing hormone; MAB=maximal androgen blockade; PSA=prostate-specific antigen long-term outcome of various treatments for localized disease. After these long-term studies are completed, important questions concerning treatments may be answered.

Conclusions

More knowledge is required for the identification of organ-confined cancer that is potentially aggressive and life-threatening, which requires prompt and curative treatment. The outcome of metastatic and hormone-refractory prostate disease remains poor, and a better understanding of their pathology is necessary.

References

Brawer MK, Chetner MP, Beatie J, Buchner DM, Vessella RL, Lange PH (1992) Screening for prostate carcinoma with prostate-specific antigen. *J Urol* **147**: 841–5

Burton JL, Oakley A, Anderson JB (2000) Recent advances in the histopathology and molecular biology of prostate cancer. *Br J Urol Int* **85**: 87–94

Carter BS, Bova GS, Beaty TH *et al* (1993) Hereditary prostate cancer: epidemiologic and clinical features. *J Urol* **150**(3): 797–802

Dearnaley DP, Kirby RS, Kirk D, Malone P, Simpson RJ, Williams G (1999) Diagnosis and management of early prostate cancer. Report of a British Association of Urological Surgeons Working Party. *Br J Urol Int* **83**: 18–33

Gerber GS, Thisted RA, Scardino PT *et al* (1996) Results of radical prostatectomy in men with clinically localized prostate cancer. *JAMA* **276**: 615–19

Gleason DF (1992) Histologic grading of prostate cancer: a perspective. *Hum Pathol* **23**: 273–9

John EM, Whittemore AS, Wu AH *et al* (1995) Vasectomy and prostate cancer: results from a multi-ethnic case-control study. *J Natl Cancer Inst* **87**: 662–9

Lee F, Patel HRH, Emberton M (2002) The 'top ten' urological procedures: a study of the hospital episodes statistics 1998–99. *Br J Urol Int* **90**: 1

Littrup PJ, Bailey SE (2000) Prostate cancer. The role of transrectal ultrasound and its impact on cancer detection and management. *Radiol Clin North Am* **38**: 87–113

Lu-Yao GL, Yao SL (1997) Population-based study of long-term survival in patients with clinically localised prostate cancer. *Lancet* **349**: 906–10

Majeed FA, Burgess NA (1994) Trends in death rates and registration rates for prostate cancer in England and Wales. *Br J Urol Int* **73**: 377–81

Murphy GP (1999) Review of phase-II hormone-refractory prostate cancer trials. *Urology* **54**: 19–21

National Statistics Office (2002) StatBase dataset. National Statistics Office, London. Available at: http://www.statistics.gov.uk/statbase/xsdataset.asp?vlnk=3352&B4.x=35&B4.y=8 Accessed 9 July 2002

Partin AW, Mangold LA, Lamm DM, Walsh PC, Epstein JI, Pearson JD (2001) Contemporary update of prostate cancer staging nomograms (Partin tables) for the new millennium. *Urology* **58**: 843–8

Prostate Cancer Trialists Collaborative Group (2000) Maximum androgen blockade in advanced prostate cancer: an overview of the randomised trials. *Lancet* **355**: 1491–8

Rietbergen JB, Kruger AE, Kranse R, Schroder FH (1997) Complications of transrectal ultrasound-guided systematic sextant biopsies of the prostate: evaluation of complication rates and risk factors within a population-based screening program. *Urology* **49**: 875–80

Smith DS, Catalona WJ (1995) Interexaminer variability of digital rectal examination in detecting prostate cancer. *Urology* **45**: 70–4

Smith RA, von Eschenbach AC, Wender R (2001) American Cancer Society guidelines for the early detection of cancer. Update of early detection guidelines for prostate, colorectal and endometrial cancers. *CA Cancer J Clin* **51**: 38–44

van der Cruijsen-Koeter IW, Wildhagen MF, de Koning HJ, Schroder FH (2001) The value of current diagnostic tests in prostate cancer screening. *Br J Urol Int* **88**: 458–66

Wiley EL, Davidson P, McIntire DD, Sagalowsky AI (1997) Risk of concurrent prostate cancer in cystoprostatectomy specimens is related to volume of high-grade prostatic intraepithelial neoplasia. *Urology* **49**: 692–6

Key points

⌘ The diagnosis of prostate cancer is made from history, examination and investigations.

⌘ Improvements in the detection of prostate cancer include prostate-specific antigen (PSA) testing and transrectal ultrasound-guided biopsy of the prostate. These enable the detection of the disease at an early stage when it is organ-confined and amenable to curative treatment.

⌘ To improve PSA sensitivity and specificity, PSA density, PSA velocity, age-related PSA and the free/total PSA ratio have been used. All increase the accuracy of diagnosing cancer, but the last method appears to be the most promising.

⌘ There are three treatment options for early (localized) prostate cancer: watchful waiting, radical radiotherapy and radical prostatectomy. The selection of treatment option is not evidence-based, but is derived from informed choices made by patients and their relatives, with assistance from the clinician.

⌘ It has been found in several studies that early androgen suppression in patients with asymptomatic metastatic disease is associated with less progression and fewer complications such as ureteric obstruction or pathological fracture.

⌘ The outcome of metastatic and hormone-refractory prostate disease remains poor, and a better understanding of their pathology is necessary.

3

Update on bladder cancer

*Shikohe Masood, Hassan Wazait, Manit Arya
and Hitendra RH Patel*

*Ten thousand new cases of bladder cancer are reported
each year in the UK. Earlier diagnosis and better care
have improved survival rates, but the incidence is still
rising. This chapter updates the current understanding of
the diagnosis and management of bladder cancer.*

Introduction

Bladder cancer is the second commonest cancer of the
genitourinary tract, and the fifth most common malignancy in
Europe (Jensen *et al*, 1990). The annual incidence in the UK is
34.0 (male) and 13.3 (female) per 100 000 population (Office for
National Statistics, 1998). Caucasians are at highest risk, with an
average age at diagnosis of sixty-five years. At the time of
diagnosis most bladder cancer is organ confined, but up to 25% of
cases will have muscle invasion or nodal disease (Waters, 1996).

Bladder cancer commonly presents with painless gross
haematuria, but can be associated with other symptoms or signs
(*Table 3.1*). Rarely, systemic disturbances occur during
presentation of advanced disease, but generally bladder cancer has
no signs at the time of diagnosis.

Table 3.1: Presenting features of bladder cancer

Features	Frequency
Painless gross haematuria	90%
Microscopic haematuria	10%
Urinary symptoms: frequency, urgency, dysuria	25%
Systemic symptoms (bone pain or acute renal failure)	Rare

Risk factors

The most common risk factor for bladder cancer is cigarette smoking, which is thought to cause bladder cancer in 50% of men and 30% of women (Wynder and Goldsmith, 1977). People working in certain industries (eg. those involving dyes, chemicals, printing, rubber, petroleum and leather) are also at high risk of bladder cancer (Matanoski and Elliot, 1981). Risk factors for bladder cancer are summarized in *Table 3.2.*

Pathology

Transitional cell carcinoma accounts for 90% and squamous cell carcinoma accounts for 5–10% of all bladder cancer in the Western world (Jensen et al, 1990; *Table 3.3*). Squamous cell carcinoma is associated with schistosomiasis, which is endemic in Africa and the Middle East, accounting for 60–70% of bladder cancer (El-Bolkainy *et al*, 1981).

Table 3.2: Risk factors for bladder cancer	
Factor	**Example**
Cigarette smoking	Multiple carcinogens
Occupational exposure	2-naphthylamine, benzidine, 4-aminobiphenyl
Dietary factors	Caffeine, artificial sweeteners (controversial)
Drugs	Cyclophosphamide, phenacetin
Chronic infections	Schistosomiasis, indwelling catheters
Chromosomal changes	Alteration in tumour-suppressor genes p53 and retinoblastoma gene
Radiotherapy	For cervical cancer and thyroid cancer

Staging and grading

Bladder cancer can be broadly divided into superficial (<pT2) and muscle-invasive tumours (≥pT2). The tumour (primary), nodes, metastasis (TNM) staging system classification (Union Internationale Contre le Cancer, 1997) enables estimation of the prognosis and selection of appropriate treatment. The pathological grade predicts recurrence, invasion and progression. Overall prognosis is estimated using both factors (*Table 3.4*).

Table 3.3: Pathological classification of bladder tumours

	Type	Frequency
Benign	Papilloma	<2%
Malignant	Transitional cell carcinoma	90%
	Squamous cell carcinoma	5–10% (Western world)
		60–70% (Middle East/Africa)
	Adenocarcinoma	<2%
	Undifferentiated	<2%
	Mixed carcinoma	4–6%
	Epithelial/non-epithelial	Rare

Table 3.4: Five-year survival rate following cystectomy

Pathological stage	5-year survival
Superficial disease	78–91%
Invasive disease	20–80%

From Stein (2000)

Management

Figure 3.1 summarizes the investigations and treatments for superficial and invasive bladder cancer.

Urine

Urine cytology shows malignant cells, especially in high-grade tumours. Other urine tests include bladder tumour antigen (Sarosdy *et al*, 1997) and nuclear matrix protein 22 (NMP22) (Soloway *et al*, 1996), which detect exfoliated markers. These tests should not be performed in the initial evaluation of haematuria, but should be reserved for use in patients after diagnosis of bladder cancer.

Imaging

Ultrasound and intravenous urogram can detect bladder cancer and upper tract abnormalities. Computed tomography scan or magnetic resonance imaging and nuclear bone scan are performed to stage bladder cancer.

Cystoscopy

The best way to diagnose a bladder cancer is via cystoscopy (rigid or flexible).

Treatment

Figure 3.1 shows the treatment options for muscle-invasive bladder cancer; treatment of superficial (non-muscle-invasive) bladder cancer is summarized below, including local intravesical therapy.

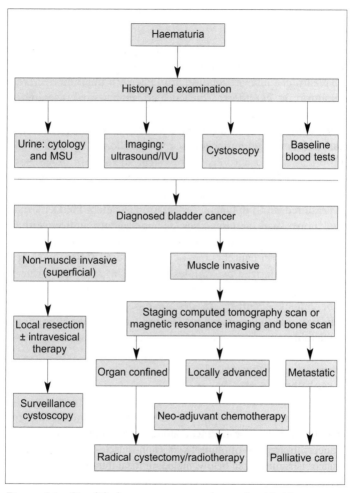

Figure 3.1: Simplified management pathway for bladder cancer. IVU=intravenous urogram; MSU=midstream urine specimen.

Superficial cancer

Patients diagnosed with a low grade, single tumour can be treated by transurethral resection followed by surveillance. The chances of recurrence and progression are high with multiple, recurrent tumours or carcinoma *in situ*, so intravesical therapy is recommended after tumour resection.

Intravesical therapy. Between 50–70% of superficial bladder cancer recurs after initial endoscopic resection (Rogerson, 1994). In order to prevent this, intravesical therapy is given post-resection. Many studies have shown that intravesical therapy reduces recurrence of the tumour, but none has shown evidence of definite reduction in tumour progression (Amling, 2001).

Intravesical therapy uses several agents (mitomycin C, thiotepa, adriamycin and doxorubicin), with limited side-effects. The immunotherapeutic agent bacille Calmette-Guérin (BCG), popularized by Morales *et al* (1976), also has a role to play. The side-effects can be striking, with systemic tuberculosis occurring in certain cases (Steg *et al*, 1989); however, in modern use these are limited. BCG has been shown to be more effective against carcinoma *in situ* (Rogerson, 1994).

Muscle-invasive tumours

Transurethral resection cannot completely remove muscle-invasive bladder tumours; it only helps in diagnosing and staging the muscle-invasive disease. Similarly, intravesical chemotherapy or immunotherapy has no role in invasive disease. For the past fifty years, definitive treatment of muscle-invasive bladder tumours has consisted of either radical cystectomy or external beam radiotherapy. Among British urologists there was a reluctance to perform radical surgery

(Hendry, 1986), and radiotherapy was preferred. Improvements in anaesthetic techniques, postoperative care and better knowledge of pelvic anatomy have caused a resurgence in radical surgery.

After surgery the urine is diverted via ileal conduit, orthotopic bladder reconstruction or continent urinary diversion. This requires follow-up, as patients can have systemic (metabolic) and local problems.

Role of chemotherapy

Chemotherapy can be given before cystectomy (neo-adjuvant) (Kolaczyk *et al*, 2002) or after radical treatment (adjuvant). At the time of diagnosis, 15% of patients with bladder cancer have disease in the lymph nodes or distant metastasis. After cystectomy and bilateral pelvic lymphadenectomy, 20–35% of patients are found to have lymph nodes affected by the cancer. Without treatment the survival is limited. Randomized, prospective trials are under way to establish the role of neo-adjuvant chemotherapy, but the follow-up period is still too limited to draw any firm conclusions.

The commonly used chemotherapy agents are cisplatin, methotrexate, doxorubicin, vinblastine, cyclophosphamide and 5-fluorouracil. Following cystectomy, patients at high risk of systemic relapse because of lymph node metastasis or regionally advanced disease are candidates for adjuvant chemotherapy (Skinner *et al*, 1991).

Follow-up

After resection of superficial bladder cancer the patient is followed-up cystoscopically to detect early recurrence. This is done initially every three months for two years, six-monthly for the next three years and then annually for life, assuming no recurrence occurs.

Patients with treated invasive bladder cancer require monitoring of areas where transitional cell epithelium remains (kidneys, ureters) by imaging and endoscopy. Cystoscopy is required in orthotopic reconstruction as there is a potential risk of adenocarcinoma within the bowel epithelium, or recurrent transitional cell carcinoma in post-radiotherapy bladders.

Recent advances

Currently, histological methods may not reliably predict the behaviour of bladder cancer. Profiling the disease at the cellular and molecular level may help improve this situation and thus enable tailored treatment. Current markers being developed include blood group-related antigens (ABH and Lewis antigen), microvessel density, retinoblastoma and p53 genes (Stein *et al*, 1998).

Intravesical therapy for high-risk patients or patients who fail first-line therapy are being developed. These agents include alpha-interferon (Belldegrun *et al*, 1998), bropiramine (Sarosdy *et al*, 1998) and AD-32 (Greenberg *et al*, 1997).

Conclusions

Early detection of bladder cancer is essential to improve survival. Improving the public's perception and healthcare professionals' awareness of this is as important as reducing environmental exposure to carcinogenic factors. Future molecular profiling to predict the behaviour of bladder cancer will hopefully improve the efficacy of treatment.

References

Amling CL (2001) Diagnosis and management of superficial bladder cancer. *Curr Probl Cancer* **25**(4): 224–78

Belldegrun AS, Franklin JR, O'Donnell MA *et al* (1998) Superficial bladder cancer: the role of interferon-alpha. *J Urol* **159**(6): 1793–801

El-Bolkainy MN, Mokhtar NM, Ghoneim MA, Hussein MH (1981) The impact of schistosomiasis on the pathology of bladder carcinoma. *Cancer* **48**: 2643

Greenberg RE, Bahnson RR, Wood D *et al* (1997) Initial report on intravesical administration of N-trifluoroacetyladriamycin-14-valerate (AD 32) to patients with refractory superficial transitional cell carcinoma of the urinary bladder. *Urology* **49**(3): 471–5

Hendry WF (1986) Morbidity and mortality of radical cystectomy (1971–1978 and 1978–1985). *J Roy Soc Med* **79**: 395–400

Jensen OM, Estere J, Muller J, Renerd H (1990) Cancer in the European community and its member states. *Eur J Cancer* **26**: 1167–77

Kolaczyk W, Dembowski J, Lorenz J, Dudek K (2002) Evaluation of the influence of systemic neoadjuvant chemotherapy on the survival of patients treated for invasive bladder cancer. *Br J Urol Int* **89**(6): 616–19

Matanoski GM, Elliot EA (1981) Bladder cancer epidemiology. *Epidemiol Rev* **3**: 203

Morales A, Eidenger D, Bruce AW (1976) Intracavitary bacille Calmette-Guérin in the treatment of superficial bladder tumours. *J Urol* **116**: 180–3

Office for National Statistics (1998) *Registration of Cancer Diagnosed in 1992.* England and Wales. Series MBI. No 25. Her Majesty's Stationery Office, London

Rogerson JW (1994) Intravesical bacille Calmette-Guérin in the treatment of superficial transitional cell carcinoma of the bladder. *Br J Urol* **73**: 655–8

Sarosdy MF, Hudson MA, Ellis WJ *et al* (1997) Improved detection of recurrent bladder cancer using the BARD BTA stat test. *Urology* **50**(3): 349–53

Sarosdy MF, Manyak MJ, Sagalowsky AI *et al* (1998) Oral bropirimine immunotherapy of bladder carcinoma *in situ* after prior intravesical bacille Calmette-Guérin. *Urology* **51**(2): 226–31

Skinner DG, Daniels JR, Russell CA *et al* (1991) The role of adjuvant chemotherapy following cystectomy for invasive bladder cancer: a prospective comparative trial. *J Urol* **145**(3): 459–64

Soloway MS, Briggman JV, Carpinto GA *et al* (1996) Use of a new tumour marker, urinary NMP-22, in the detection of occult or rapidly recurring transitional cell carcinoma of the urinary tract following surgical treatment. *J Urol* **156**: 363–7

Steg A, Leleu C, Debre B, Boccon-Gibod L, Sicard D (1989) Systemic bacillus Calmette-Guérin infection in patients treated by intravesical BCG therapy for superficial bladder cancer. *Prog Clin Biol Res* **310**: 325–34

Stein JP (2000) Indications of early cystectomy. *Semin Urol Oncol* **18**(4): 289–95

Stein JP, Grossfeld GD, Ginsberg DA *et al* (1998) Prognostic markers in bladder cancer: a contemporary review of the literature. *J Urol* **160**: 645–59

Union Internationale Contre le Cancer (1997) Bladder cancer. In: Sobin LH, Wittekind C, eds. *TNM Classification of Malignant Tumours*. 5th edn. Wiley-Liss, New York: 309–14

Waters WB (1996) Invasive bladder cancer – where do we go from here? *J Urol* **155**(6): 1910–11

Wynder EL, Goldsmith K (1977) The epidemiology of bladder cancer: a second look. *Cancer* **40**: 1246

Key points

- ⌘ Bladder cancer is the second commonest cancer of the genitourinary tract, and the fifth most common malignancy in Europe, with 10 000 new cases reported each year in the UK.

- ⌘ Bladder cancer commonly presents with painless gross haematuria, but can be associated with other symptoms or signs, such as microscopic haematuria, urinary symptoms and, rarely, systemic symptoms.

- ⌘ The most common risk factor for bladder cancer is cigarette smoking, which is thought to cause bladder cancer in 50% of men and 30% of women.

- ⌘ Bladder cancer can be broadly divided into superficial (<pT2) and muscle-invasive tumours (≥pT2).

- ⌘ Patients diagnosed with a low grade, single tumour can be treated by transurethral resection followed by surveillance.

- ⌘ For the past 50 years, definitive treatment of muscle-invasive bladder tumours has consisted of either radical cystectomy or external beam radiotherapy. Chemotherapy can be given before cystectomy (neo-adjuvant) or after radical treatment (adjuvant).

- ⌘ Early detection of bladder cancer is essential to improve survival. Improving the public's perception and healthcare professionals' awareness of this is as important as reducing environmental exposure to carcinogenic factors.

4

Kidney cancer: management guidelines

Frank Lee and Hitendra RH Patel

Renal cell carcinoma accounts for 2% of all cancers. Medical progress has improved the outcome of early but not advanced disease. This chapter highlights the current practice for the management of renal cell carcinoma.

Introduction

Renal cell carcinoma (RCC) is known as the 'physician's tumour' because of its wide range of presenting characteristics (*Table 4.1*) and associated systemic disturbances (*Table 4.2*). Awareness of these features among cross-specialty practitioners avoids diagnostic delay by prompt investigation and referral, thus improving patient outcome.

Epidemiology

Two per cent of all adult malignancies are RCC, with the highest incidence occurring in patients in their seventies (median=66 years). Hellsten *et al* (1990) reported a 2% incidence of RCC at autopsy from all causes of death in a single institution.

Table 4.1: Relative frequency of presenting features in patients with renal cell carcinoma

Features	Relative frequency
Pain	1 in 3
Haematuria	1 in 3
Weight loss	1 in 3
Mass	1 in 5
Hypertension	1 in 5
Fever	1 in 5
Classic triad	1 in 10
Hypercalcaemia	1 in 20

From Belldegrun and deKernion (1998)

Table 4.2: Relative frequency of systemic disturbances in patients with renal cell carcinoma

Systemic disturbance	Relative frequency
Increased erythrocyte sedimentation rate	1 in 2
Hypertension	1 in 3
Anaemia	1 in 3
Weight loss, cachexia	1 in 3
Pyrexia	1 in 10
Deranged hepatic function	1 in 10
Raised alkaline phosphatase	1 in 10
Hypercalcaemia	1 in 20
Polycythaemia	<1 in 20
Neuromyopathy	<1 in 20
Amyloidosis	<1 in 20

From Chisholm (1974)

More men are affected than women (2:1 respectively), with RCC being the eighth commonest cancer in men and the fourteenth in women (Office for National Statistics, 1996a,b). In 1996, there were 3450 new cases of kidney cancer in men and 2160 cases in women (Office for National Statistics, 1996a,b). The incidence of RCC increased from 13% in 1973 to 61% in 1998 (Jayson and Sanders, 1998), mainly because of the rising number of incidental tumours detected by either ultrasound or computed tomography (CT) imaging in asymptomatic patients being investigated for other intra-abdominal pathology.

Pathology

Each anatomical element in the kidney can give rise to benign and malignant tumours (*Table 4.3*). RCC is believed to originate from the proximal renal tubular cells, with most being unilateral. Bilateral tumours (either synchronous or metachronous) account for 2% of cases (eg. von Hippel–Lindau disease, VHLD) (Iliopoulos and Eng, 2000).

Macroscopically, RCC are usually rounded and have a pseudocapsule composed of compressed renal parenchyma and fibrous tissue. There are areas of yellow or brown tumour interposed between patches of haemorrhage and necrosis; calcification and cystic areas may also be present. The common sites for metastasis are lung, bone, liver, adrenal and brain, occurring via the blood and lymphatic stream equally.

Histologically, RCC can be divided into subtypes of conventional (clear cell), papillary, chromophobic and multilocular cystic tumour (Storkel *et al*, 1997). All these tumour types can show cytoplasmic granularity or spindle cell features. Therefore, 'granular' and 'sarcomatoid' RCC no longer exist as distinct entities in the latest classification.

Table 4.3: Pathological classification of some renal tumours

Benign	Simple cyst		
	Angiomyolipoma		
	Oncocytoma		
	Phaeochromocytoma		
	Leiomyoma		
	Haemangioma		
	Fibroma		
	Arteriovenous malformation		
Malignant	Primary	Renal cell carcinoma	
		Liposarcoma	
		Leiomyosarcoma	
		Rhabdomyosarcoma	
	Metastatic	Local	Adrenal
		Distant	Carcinoid
			Leukaemia
			Lymphoma

Risk factors

Environmental factors

Smoking (cigarette, cigar and pipe), obesity, a high protein diet and exposure to petrol, cadmium and lead have been postulated as risk factors for RCC (Dhote *et al*, 2000).

Genetic factors

Familial forms of papillary and clear cell RCC exist. However, the discovery of the von Hippel–Lindau gene (chromosome 3p) associated with VHLD has improved our understanding of the genetic basis of RCC (Iliopoulos and Eng, 2000). Other oncogenes implicated include erbB, c-myc and tuberous sclerosis-2 tumour-suppressor genes (Kirkali et al, 2001). In this whole group, 35–40% of patients will die of RCC if early detection and treatment does not occur.

Other factors

Hypertension, diuretics and renal stones have been suggested as risk factors for RCC (Dhote *et al*, 2000). Malignant change can also occur within acquired renal cysts secondary to long-term dialysis (Brennan *et al*, 1991; Sant and Ucci, 1998).

Clinical presentation

The classic triad of haematuria, loin pain and a mass is found in only 10% of patients and is suggestive of advanced disease (*Table 4.1*). The most common presentation is 'incidental'. However, 25–30% of patients have metastatic disease at the time of presentation (Motzer *et al*, 1997).

Hypertension can be caused by segmental renal artery occlusion or the production of renin (or renin-like) substance. Polycythaemia and hypercalcaemia (paraneoplastic syndrome) occur as a result of the production of erythropoietin and parathyroid hormone-like substance respectively. Non-metastatic hepatic dysfunction with necrosis and fever can occur (Staufer's syndrome). Persistence or recurrence of this post-nephrectomy is invariably associated with tumour recurrence.

Staging and prognosis

Staging is crucial in planning management and providing prognostic information. The tumour, node and metastasis (TNM) system was revised in 1997, reflecting the improved management of the disease and also accounting for the lack of significant survival difference between tumours <2.5 cm and those <7 cm in size (Guinan *et al*, 1997). This cut-off size has been controversial, as other dimensions have recently been proposed (eg. tumours <4 cm may be suitable for nephron-sparing surgery; Herr, 1994; Fergany *et al*, 2000; Lee *et al*, 2000).

Apart from pathological stage, important prognostic factors include tumour size (an independent factor on its own), nuclear grade and ploidy, and the performance status of the patient (Thrasher and Paulson, 1993). Some patient-related factors have been identified as having a survival impact. These include time from diagnosis to metastasis, location and number of metastases, weight loss and whether nephrectomy has been performed (Maldazys and deKernion, 1986). There are other markers currently under evaluation as potential predictors of outcome, such as nuclear morphometry, serum ferritin and molecular markers measuring tumour cell proliferation, growth factors, cell adhesion, apoptosis, telomerase activity and angiogenesis.

The five-year survival rate for patients with localized (organ-confined), locally advanced (perinephric tissue involvement with intact Gerota's fascia) and metastatic RCC are about 70–90%, 60% and 4% respectively (Chowdhury and Gore, 1999). There is a need for other treatment modalities to improve the poor outcome in metastatic RCC.

Management

Investigations

A thorough history will elucidate the risk factors mentioned earlier, and baseline investigations should include a full blood count, urea, creatinine and electrolytes, and urine for microscopy, culture, sensitivity and cytology. If haematuria is present, this should be investigated as previously described (Harper *et al*, 2001). *Figure 4.1* gives a management algorithm once a renal mass is located.

Treatment

Surgery is the only curative treatment in localized RCC. Radical nephrectomy is still the gold standard in the presence of a normal contralateral kidney. However, evidence suggests that partial nephrectomy is equally safe in organ-confined tumours (≤4 cm in size; Herr, 1994; Fergany *et al*, 2000; Lee *et al*, 2000). Thus, it can be offered to patients with a solitary kidney, a functionally compromised contralateral kidney or in bilateral RCC.

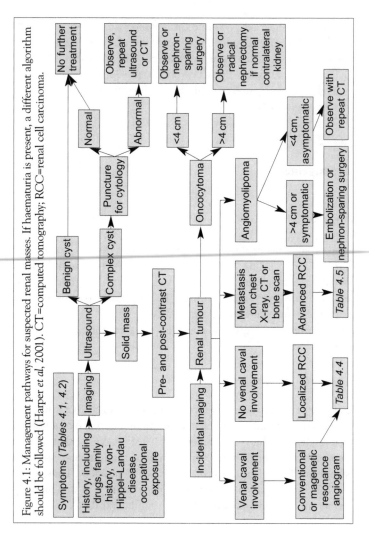

Figure 4.1: Management pathways for suspected renal masses. If haematuria is present, a different algorithm should be followed (Harper *et al*, 2001). CT=computed tomography; RCC=renal cell carcinoma.

At present, there is no cure for advanced RCC. Cytotoxic and hormonal therapies are of limited use. Radiotherapy is only used for the symptomatic treatment of bone or cerebral metastases. Patients with solitary metastasis may be considered for nephrectomy and excision of the metastatic lesion, but limited evidence exists for outcome.

In patients with advanced disease, alpha-interferon has a 15–20% response rate (Belldegrun and deKernion, 1998). Recombinant interleukin-2 therapy has shown more success in terms of a higher response rate and a longer remission time. With regard to the role of cytoreductive nephrectomy in conjunction with immunotherapy, two prospective studies have shown a beneficial effect and that nephrectomy before immunotherapy is superior to immunotherapy alone (Flanigan *et al*, 1999; Mickisch *et al*, 1999).

Table 4.4: Treatment options for localized renal cell carcinoma

Localized	≤4 cm or solitary functioning kidney	Radical nephrectomy with subsequent renal substitution therapy, e.g. dialysis
		Nephron-sparing surgery (open or laparoscopic)
	>4 cm with normal contralateral kidney	Radical nephrectomy
Localized with supra-diaphragmatic caval involvement	Same as management of localized disease but requires cardiothoracic consult and support, e.g. cardiopulmonary bypass	
Locally advanced	Radical nephrectomy	

Follow-up

There is no consensus or published guidelines at present, but follow-up should be coordinated via a multidisciplinary team. The interval and the performance of physical examination, serum bone profile, chest X-ray and abdominal CT are tailored to the pathological stage, the individual patient's wishes (eg. regular review for reassurance *vs* 'prefer not to know') and the knowledge that survival may not be prolonged by the early detection of tumour recurrence.

Table 4.5: Treatment options for advanced renal cell carcinoma

Solitary metastasis	Radical nephrectomy and excision of metastatic lesion	
	Manage as for multiple metastases	
Multiple metastases	Enter into clinical trial for immunotherapy	
	Palliative, symptomatic treatment of bone pain, cerebral oedema, renal pain, intractable haematuria	Non-steroidal anti-inflammatory, opiate
		Palliative radiotherapy
		Steroids and radiotherapy
		Embolization
		Nephrectomy

On the horizon

Gene therapy using transformed autologous tumour cells, tumour infiltrating lymphocytes or encoding of the major histocompatibility complex class I molecules has demonstrated a reduction in tumour growth, metastasis and rejection of subsequent tumour challenges in a murine model (Figlin, 1999). Likewise, monoclonal therapy against the carbonic anhydrase IX antigen in clear cell carcinoma of the kidney has shown excellent targeting results in mice (Lampe and Oosterwijk, 2000). Thus, tumour cell targeting with cytotoxic agents is possible. Researchers have also demonstrated the possibility of using dendritic cells in a RCC vaccine in patients (Kugler *et al*, 2000).

Conclusions

There have been improvements in the diagnosis, staging, management and survival in patients with localized RCC. Unfortunately, the outlook for advanced disease remains poor, although a better understanding of RCC tumour biology may help improve the outcome in these patients.

References

Belldegrun A, deKernion JB (1998) Renal tumors. In: Retik AB, Vaughan ED Jr, Walsh PC, Wein AJ, eds. *Campbell's Urology*. 7th edn. WB Saunders, Philadelphia: 2299

Brennan JF, Stilmant MM, Babayan RK, Siroky MB (1991) Acquired renal cystic disease: implications for the urologist. *Br J Urol* **67**(4): 342–8

Chisholm GD (1974) Nephrogenic ridge tumors and their syndromes. *Ann N Y Acad Sci* **230**: 403–23

Chowdhury S, Gore M (1999) The management of metastatic renal cell carcinoma. *Urol Cancer Abstr* **4**: 2–5

Dhote R, Pellicer-Coeuret M, Thiounn N, Debre B, Vidal-Trecan G (2000) Risk factors for adult renal cell carcinoma: a systematic review and implications for prevention. *Br J Urol Int* **86**(1): 20–7

Fergany AF, Hafez KS, Novick AC (2000) Long-term results of nephron-sparing surgery for localized renal cell carcinoma: 10-year follow-up. *J Urol* **163**(2): 442–5

Figlin RA (1999) Renal cell carcinoma: management of advanced disease. *J Urol* **161**(2): 381–6

Flanigan RC, Salmon SE, Blumstein BA (1999) Cytoreductive nephrectomy in metastatic renal cell carcinoma: the results of Southwest Oncology Group (SWOG) trial 8949. *J Urol* (suppl) **163**: 154 (abstract 685)

Guinan P, Sobin LH, Algaba F *et al* (1997) TNM staging of renal cell carcinoma: workgroup No.3. Union International Contre Le Cancer (UICC) and the American Joint Committee on Cancer (AJCC). *Cancer* **80**(5): 992–3

Harper M, Arya M, Hamid R, Patel HRH (2001) Haematuria: a streamlined approach to management. *Hosp Med* **62**(11): 696–8

Hellsten S, Johnsen J, Berge T, Linell F (1990) Clinically unrecognized renal cell carcinoma. Diagnostic and pathological aspects. *Eur Urol* **18**(suppl 2): 2–3

Herr HW (1994) Partial nephrectomy for incidental renal cell carcinoma. *Br J Urol* **74**(4): 431–3

Iliopoulos O, Eng C (2000) Genetic and clinical aspects of familial renal neoplasms. *Semin Oncol* **27**(2): 138–49

Jayson M, Sanders H (1998) Increased incidence of serendipitously discovered renal cell carcinoma. *Urology* **51**(2): 203–5

Kirkali Z, Tuzel E, Mungan MU (2001) Recent advances in kidney cancer and metastatic disease. *Br J Urol Int* **88**(8): 818–24

Kugler A, Stuhler G, Walden P *et al* (2000) Regression of human metastatic renal cell carcinoma after vaccination with tumor cell-dendritic cell hybrids. *Nat Med* **6**(3): 332–6

Lampe MI, Oosterwijk E (2000) New developments in the use of monoclonal antibodies in the therapy of genitourinary cancer. *Br J Urol Int* **86**(2): 165–71

Lee CT, Katz J, Shi W, Thaler HT, Reuter VE, Russo P (2000) Surgical management of renal tumors 4 cm or less in a contemporary cohort. *J Urol* **163**(3): 730–6

Maldazys JD, deKernion JB (1986) Prognostic factors in metastatic renal carcinoma. *J Urol* **136**(2): 376–9

Mickisch GH, Garin A, Madej M (1999) Tumor nephrectomy plus interferon alpha is superior to interferon alpha alone in metastatic renal cell carcinoma. *J Urol* **163**(suppl): 176(abstract 778)

Motzer RJ, Russo P, Nanus DM, Berg WJ (1997) Renal cell carcinoma. *Curr Probl Cancer* **21**(4): 185–232

Office for National Statistics (1996a) Cancer trends appendix 1: cancer incidence statistics for males, United Kingdom, 1996. Available at: http://www.statistics.gov.uk/ statbase/xsdataset.asp?vlnk=3226&B4.x=37&B4.y=16 Accessed 22 March 2002

Office for National Statistics (1996b) Cancer trends appendix 1: cancer incidence statistics for females, United Kingdom, 1996. Available at: http://www.statistics.gov.uk/statbase/xsdataset.asp?vlnk=3227&B4.x=50&B4.y=10 Accessed 22 March 2002

Sant GR, Ucci AA Jr (1998) Acquired renal cystic disease and adenocarcinoma following renal transplantation — a current urologic perspective. *Urol Int* **60**(2): 108–12

Storkel S, Eble JN, Adlakha F *et al* (1997) Classification of renal cell carcinoma: workgroup No. 1. Union Internationale Contre le Cancer (UICC) and the American Joint Committee on Cancer (AJCC). *Cancer* **80**(5): 987–9

Thrasher JB, Paulson DF (1993) Prognostic factors in renal cancer. *Urol Clin North Am* **20**(2): 247–62

Key points

- Renal cell carcinoma (RCC) is not common but can present to practitioners other than urologists because of its variety of symptoms.

- An increase in abdominal ultrasound and computed tomography has resulted in the detection of more incidental RCC with a smaller size and lower stage.

- Radical nephrectomy offers the best chance of cure in patients with localized RCC.

- There is emerging evidence that nephron-sparing surgery in patients with a localized RCC ≤4 cm does not compromise survival.

- The management of oncocytoma and angio-myolipoma is controversial. Those patients who are managed with observation should be monitored carefully, eg. with regular computed tomography.

- Immunotherapy can provide some survival benefits. A better understanding of RCC tumour biology may bring about a better response rate and duration of survival in the future.

- Improvement in the prognosis of advanced RCC is likely to rely upon future advances in gene therapy, monoclonal therapy and tumour vaccine.

5

Testicular cancer: update and controversies

Frank Lee, Manit Arya and Hitendra RH Patel

Testicular cancer is the commonest cancer in men aged twenty to thirty-four years of age. Radical orchidectomy is the conventional initial treatment, and the overall five-year survival rate has improved to 95%. However, there is room for improvement in the treatment of advanced disease, maintaining the high cure rate while reducing the associated morbidity and toxicity.

Introduction

Testicular cancer is relatively uncommon; it primarily affects young men, and the treatment of radical orchidectomy has a tremendous psychological burden on the patient. The use of serum markers to detect and monitor treatment, plus the use of platinum-based agents for metastatic disease, have resulted in an overall one-year and five-year survival rate of almost 98% and 95% respectively (Quinn *et al*, 2001). The quest is for therapeutic modalities for metastatic disease that have superior efficacy but better side-effect profiles so that the patient's quality of life, such as sexual function and fertility, can be preserved.

Epidemiology

Although testicular cancer only accounts for about 1% of all malignancies in men at all ages, it is the most common cancer in men aged between twenty and thirty-four years (Quinn *et al*, 2001); approximately 50% of all testicular cancers occur in men under thirty-five years of age. The incidence in the UK in 1996 was 1770, while there were ninety deaths from testicular cancer in 1998 (Quinn *et al*, 2001). The incidence has nearly doubled since 1971. This may be caused by endogenous or exogenous (environmental) oestrogenic compounds that affect the embryonic testis and increase the subsequent risk of carcinogenesis (Sharpe and Skakkebaek, 1993).

Risk factors

There are a number of suggested risk factors for testicular cancer (*Table 5.1*). The role of testicular microlithiasis (TM) as a risk factor has been widely debated. TM is an ultrasound appearance of:

> ... *innumerable tiny bright echoes diffusely and uniformly scattered throughout the substance of the testicle.*
> (Doherty *et al*, 1987).

TM occurs in more than 5% of healthy young men (Peterson *et al*, 2001). The same group concluded that TM is a common finding in asymptomatic men and may not be related to testicular cancer. However, opposing evidence exists where interval testicular cancer was found in 5.4% of patients during follow-up ultrasound (Otite *et al*, 2001). Since germ cell tumours develop from carcinoma *in situ* (CIS), it would be useful to diagnose testicular cancer at this early stage. Although CIS is asymptomatic, it is associated with the presence of TM. Therefore, some advocate testicular biopsy when TM is found (Holm *et al*, 2001).

Trauma and vasectomy have not been proven as risk factors. However, non-manual or professional workers have a higher incidence of testicular cancer (Quinn *et al*, 2001).

Table 5.1: Suggested risk factors for developing testicular cancer

Factor	Relative risk
Testicular maldescent	≥3.8 if orchidectomy not performed
Infantile hernia	1.9
Low birth weight	2.6
Positive family history, e.g. siblings of patients	6–10, found to be associated with Xq27 mutation (Rapley *et al*, 2000)
Geographical/ environmental/ lifestyle/genetic factors	eg. American black people have roughly 3 times less risk than American white people, but ten times more risk than African black people
In-utero exposure to oestrogen	5
Carcinoma *in situ*	50% of patients will develop testicular cancer within five years
History of contralateral testicular cancer	28
Testicular microlithiasis	Not clearly defined at present, but biopsy advocated by some (see text)

Pathology

The histopathology of testicular tumours is complex. A simplified classification is shown in *Table 5.2*, using the British sub-classification of non-seminomatous germ cell tumours (NSGCT; Pugh and Cameron, 1976).

Table 5.2: Histological classification of testicular cancer

Anatomical origin			Histological type	
Primary tumour (~50%)	Germinal elements (~90–95%)	Germ cell tumours	Seminoma	
			NSGCT (~33%)	Teratoma differentiated
				Malignant Intermediate
				Undifferentiated
				Trophoblastic
			Yolk sac tumour	
			Mixed tumours (~10%)	
	Non-germinal elements (~5%)	Non-germ tumours	Specialized gonadal stromal neoplasms	Leydig cell tumour
				Other gonadal stromal tumours
				Gonadoblastoma
				Miscellaneous tumours, eg. carcinoid
Secondary tumour		Reticuloendothelial tumours	eg. lymphoma	
		Metastases		

NSGCT=Non-seminomatous germ cell tumours

Testicular tumours metastasize via the lymphatic system (initially to the para-aortic nodes) and haematogenous routes (commoner in NSGCT, to the lungs, liver and brain).

Staging

Staging enables important management decisions to be made and provides prognostic information. With the introduction of alternative treatment protocols for low-stage disease, its accuracy and impact become even more crucial.

There are many systems in use, and an example is shown in *Table 5.3*.

Prognostic factors

Apart from staging, the International Germ Cell Cancer Collaborative Group (1997) had introduced further criteria incorporating serum markers (pre-treatment levels of alpha-fetoprotein (AFP), human chorionic gonadotrophin (hCG) and lactate dehydrogenase (LDH)) and anatomical features (the primary tumour site and the presence of non-pulmonary visceral metastases). These parameters were found to be the most important independent prognostic factors for survival in NSGCT (*Table 5.4*).

A similar table (*Table 5.5*) is shown for prognostic factors for survival in seminoma.

Table 5.3: The Royal Marsden Hospital staging system for testicular cancer

Stage	Description			
I	No evidence of metastasis	IM	Rising concentrations of serum markers without other evidence of metastasis	
II	Abdominal lymphadenopathy	A	≤2 cm in diameter	
		B	2–5 cm in diameter	
		C	≥5 cm in diameter	
III	Supradiaphragmatic lymphadenopathy	M	Mediastinal	
		N	Supraclavicular, cervical or axillary	
		0	No abdominal lymphadenopathy	
		A, B or C	Nodal status as defined in stage II	
IV	Extralymphatic metastasis	Lung	L1	≤3 metastases
			L2	≥3 metastases, all ≤2cm in diameter
			L3	≥3 metastases, one or more of which are ≥2 cm in diameter
		Liver	H+	Liver metastases
			Br+	Brain metastases
			Bo+	Bone metastases

From Horwich (1995)

Table 5.4: Prognostic groups for non-seminomatous germ cell tumours

Prognostic group (proportion of patients)	AFP (μg/ml)	hCG (IU/ml)	LDH (x normal)	Presence of non-pulmonary metastases	5-year survival rate (%)
Good (56%)	<1	<5	<1.5	No	92%
Intermediate (28%)	1–10	5–50	1.5–10	No	80%
Poor (16%)	>10	>50	>10	Yes	48%

From International Germ Cell Cancer Collaborative Group (1997). AFP=alpha-fetoprotein, hCG=human chorionic gonadotrophin, LDH=lactic acid dehydrogenase

Table 5.5: Prognostic groups for seminoma

Prognostic group (percentage of patients)	Presence of non-pulmonary metastasis	5-year survival rate (%)
Good (90%)	No	86%
Intermediate (10%)	Yes	72%

NB. No patients were classified as having a poor prognosis. From International Germ Cell Cancer Collaborative Group (1997)

Diagnosis

Diagnosis is based on history, physical examination and investigations, including histological examination after radical orchidectomy (*Figure 5.1*).

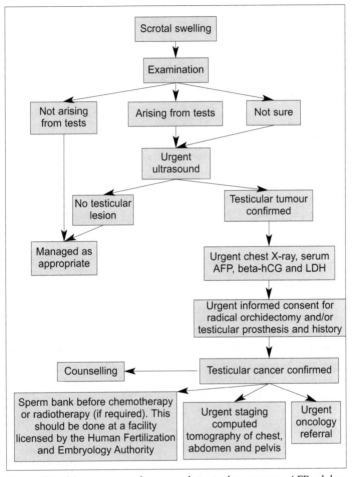

Figure 5.1: Management of suspected testicular tumour. AFP=alpha-fetoprotein; hCG=human chorionic gonadotrophin; LDH=lactic acid dehydrogenase.

History

The presenting features are summarized in *Table 5.6*.

Table 5.6: Presenting features of testicular tumour	
	Symptom
Local effects	Painless lump
	Testicular ache/discomfort
	Enlargement or firmness of testis
	Asymmetry
Metastatic effects	Back pain (para-aortic lymphadenopathy)
	Breathlessness or haemoptysis (pulmonary metastasis)

Examination

It is important to differentiate lumps arising from the testis from other intra-scrotal structures, such as the epididymis, or inguinal scrotal swellings. Patients with epididymo-orchitis or orchitis who have not improved within two weeks should be referred for an urgent urological opinion according to the Clinical Oncology Information Network (2000).

Investigations

Imaging. Ultrasound is non-invasive and can confirm a testicular lesion in most cases. Computed tomography plays an important role in the staging and follow up of patients. Positron emission tomography may have an important role in detecting residual masses after treatment of advanced disease.

Serum tumour markers. Serum tumour markers (*Table 5.7*) are important in the diagnosis, prognosis, monitoring of treatment and follow up of testicular cancer. AFP is a fetal serum-binding protein. It is normally found in minimal quantities (<100 ng/l) after the first year of life. Pure seminoma does not cause an elevation in AFP. hCG is normally produced by syncytiotrophoblasts of the placenta. Normal men have serum levels of the beta subunit of <5 mIU/ml. LDH is an enzyme responsible for lactic acid oxidation in muscle, liver and kidneys. It is useful as a marker of large volume disease and may be the only biochemical abnormality in as many as 10% of persistent or recurrent NSGCT. The reverse transcription polymerase chain reaction has enabled the differentiation of placental alkaline phosphatase from germ cell-specific alkaline phosphatase; they are elevated in NSGCT and seminoma respectively (Kommoss *et al*, 2000). Inhibin-alpha is a promising marker for Leydig cell tumours because it is absent from germ cell tumours.

Unfortunately, these markers are not specific for testicular cancer and their use should be correlated with other clinical findings.

Management

Radical orchidectomy is the conventional initial treatment of testicular cancer. This is done via an inguinal approach without breaching the scrotal skin. In patients with synchronous bilateral testicular cancer or a single testicle, an alternative of organ-sparing surgery may be considered. The feasibility of this option was shown in selected patients with organ-confined tumours of <20 mm and a normal testosterone level (Heidenreich *et al*, 2001).

Tumour marker	Elevated in
AFP	NSGCT (50–60%)
hCG	Choriocarcinoma (100%)
	Embryonal tumour (80%)
	Pure seminoma (10–25%)
LDH isoenzyme 1	Advanced or large volume
	Advanced pure seminoma
PLAP	NSGCT
GCAP	Seminoma
Inhibin-alpha	Leydig cell tumour

Table 5.7: Serum tumour markers commonly in use

AFP=alpha-fetoprotein, GCAP=germ cell-specific alkaline phosphatase, hCG=human chorionic gonadotrophin, LDH=lactic acid dehydrogenase, NSGCT=non-seminomatous germ cell tumour, PLAP=placental alkaline phosphatase

Seminoma

Although 80% of patients are cured by radical orchidectomy alone, surveillance for stage I disease is viewed by some as an investigational approach (Dearnaley *et al*, 2001) (*Figure 5.2*). This is because the conventional approach has a high success rate. Furthermore, the serum tumour markers are less reliable in detecting recurrence than in NSGCT, making follow up more difficult. In addition, recurrence may occur years after orchidectomy, but some believe that this practice is safe (Francis *et al*, 2000; Oliver, 2001).

One difficult problem regarding advanced seminoma after chemotherapy is the lack of complete resolution of radiographical masses. Surgical resection of such masses is difficult because seminoma involves the retroperitoneum in a fibrotic process similar to retroperitoneal fibrosis. Clean dissection is rarely possible, but if the residual mass is ≥3 cm, a viable tumour is found in about 50% of patients (Motzer *et al*, 1987). Hence surgical resection is advisable in this group.

NSGCT

Based on clinical trial results, a strict surveillance protocol was established for the low-risk group in stage I disease, with chemotherapy reserved for the 30% of patients who developed metastasis (Read *et al*, 1992) (*Figure 5.3*). The frequency of surveillance computed tomography is currently under review. Alternatively, adjuvant chemotherapy (two courses) could be administered immediately in the high-risk group (Cullen, 1996). With either approach, the overall survival is nearly 100%.

About one third of patients with stage II–IV disease will have residual para-aortic masses after chemotherapy. About 10% of these masses will have active undifferentiated malignant tumours. The remaining masses will contain differentiated teratoma or necrotic and fibrotic tissue. The former is unstable and is probably responsible for the late relapses. Resection of all of these masses is therefore recommended.

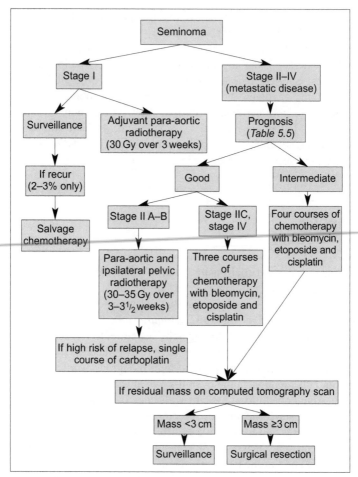

Figure 5.2: Suggested management of seminoma after radical orchidectomy and staging. The actual regimen may vary according to local expertise, opinion and protocol.

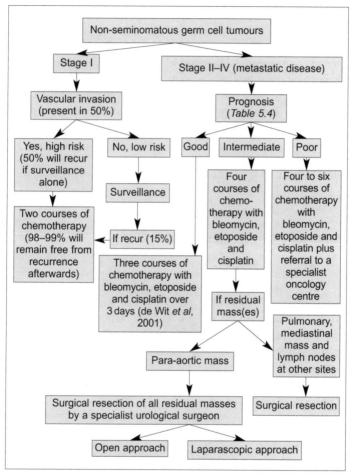

Figure 5.3: Suggested management for non-seminomatous germ cell tumours after radical orchidectomy and staging. The actual regimen may vary according to local expertise, opinion and protocol.

Persistent disease

About 15% of patients will not be cured despite a combination of therapy and surgery (Dearnaley *et al*, 2001), which poses a challenging management problem. A combination of high-dose chemotherapy with stem cell support, surgical resection and occasionally radiotherapy can be used, achieving a cure in about 30% of men (Horwich, 1995).

Side effects of treatment

Chemotherapy

These side effects are summarized in *Table 5.8*.

Surgery

Retroperitoneal lymph node dissection can cause infertility as a result of either failure of any seminal emission or retrograde ejaculation secondary to damage to the sympathetic fibres involved in ejaculation. However, the modification and improvement in surgical technique has enabled the return of ejaculation in 50–90% of patients after surgery, depending on the side and stage of the tumour (Horwich, 1995).

Follow up

Follow up is an integral part of the management of patients with testicular cancer. Apart from monitoring the effect of treatment, detecting contralateral cancer, treatment-related toxicity and relapse at an early stage when salvage treatment is still effective, it provides support and counselling to patients and their partners.

While a regimen had been described in the Clinical Oncology Information Network of the Royal College of Radiologists (2002), the optimum timing for clinical and radiological follow up is still controversial. It has been suggested that all patients with seminoma and those with stage I NSGCT may be discharged five years after treatment (Dearnaley *et al*, 2001). However, patients with metastatic NSGCT continue to have an annual relapse rate of 1–2%, even after ten years. Dearnaley *et al* (2001) also suggested that longer term follow up is necessary.

Follow up by a specialist centre has the advantages of a multidisciplinary team approach, access to databases of large numbers of patients, and the possibility of auditing results. However, this may not be convenient for all patients, and follow up by GPs with an interest in this area and easy access to the specialist centre may be an alternative.

On the horizon

Experimental prognostic factors

Experimental prognostic factors are summarized in *Table 5.9*, although more research is required to prove their value.

Clinical trials

For seminoma, trials are being conducted to assess whether the dose of radiation can be reduced to 20 Gy for stage I disease, and to assess the use of carboplatin as a single agent. For NSGCT, studies are underway to investigate new agents such as paclitaxel, 'dose-intense' schedules using weekly treatment and high-dose treatment with stem-cell rescue for patients with a poor prognosis. Efforts are being made in search of a less toxic, platinum-based regimen, and the use of vanadium-containing agents is being studied (Ghosh *et al*, 2000).

Table 5.8: Side-effects of chemotherapy

Short term	Nausea and vomiting	
	Fatigue	
	Alopecia	
	Neutropenia and sepsis	
	Nephropathy	
Long term	From bleomycin	Pulmonary toxicity
		Changes in skin pigmentation and nails
		Raynaud's syndrome
	From cisplatin	Peripheral and auditory nerve neuropathy
		Avascular necrosis of the hip
	Azoospermia (irreversible in 20–30% of patients)	
	Second malignancy, eg. leukaemia. This risk applies to both chemotherapy and radiotherapy (Travis *et al*, 2000)	
	Increase in cardiac events (Meinardi *et al*, 2000)	

Table 5.9: Experimental prognostic factors	
Marker	
Cell proliferation markers (Moul *et al*, 1993)	DNA index
	S-phase fraction
	Proliferation index
Molecular markers (Bosl *et al*, 1989)	Isochromosome 12p
Proto-oncogene (Strohmeyer *et al*, 1991)	hst-1

Conclusions

Although the overall survival rate for testicular cancer is good, there is still room for improvement in the treatment of advanced disease, maintaining the high cure rate while reducing the associated morbidity and toxicity.

References

Bosl GJ, Dmitrovsky E, Reuter VE *et al* (1989) Isochromosome of the short arm of chromosome 12: clinically useful markers for male germ cell tumors. *J Natl Cancer Inst* **81**: 1874–8

Clinical Oncology Information Network (2000) Guidelines on the management of adult testicular cancer. *Clin Oncol* **12**(suppl): 173–210

Cullen MH (1996) Adjuvant chemotherapy in high-risk stage I non-seminomatous germ cell tumours of the testis. In: Horwich A, ed. *Testicular Cancer – Investigation and Management*. Chapman and Hall, London: 181–91

Dearnaley D, Huddart R, Horwich A (2001) Managing testicular cancer. *Br Med J* **322**: 1583–8 de Wit R, Roberts JT, Wilkinson PM *et al* (2001) Equivalence of three or four cycles of bleomycin, etoposide and cisplatin chemotherapy and of a 3- or 5-day schedule in good-prognosis germ cell cancer: a randomized study of the European Organization for Research and Treatment of Cancer Genitourinary Tract Cancer Cooperative Group and the Medical Research Council. *J Clin Oncol* **19**: 1629–40

Doherty FJ, Mullins TL, Sant GR, Drinkwater MA, Ucci AA Jr (1987) Testicular microlithiasis. A unique sonographic appearance. *J Ultrasound Med* **6**: 389–92

Francis R, Bower M, Brunstrom G et al (2000) Surveillance for stage I testicular germ cell tumours: results and cost–benefit analysis of management options. *Eur J Cancer* **36**: 1925–32

Ghosh P, D'Cruz OJ, Narla RK, Uckun FM (2000) Apoptosis-inducing vanadocene compounds against human testicular cancer. *Clin Cancer Res* **6**: 1536–45

Heidenreich A, Weissbach L, Holtl W et al (2001) Organ-sparing surgery for malignant germ cell tumor of the testis. *J Urol* **166**: 2161–5

Holm M, Lenz S, De Meyts ER, Skakkebaek NE (2001) Microcalcifications and carcinoma *in situ* of the testis. *Br J Urol Int* **87**: 144–9

Horwich A (1995) Testicular cancer. In: Horwich A, ed. *Oncology — a Multidisciplinary Textbook*. Chapman and Hall, London: 485–98

International Germ Cell Cancer Collaborative Group (1997) International germ cell consensus classification: a prognostic factor-based staging system for metastatic germ cell cancers. *J Clin Oncol* **15**: 594–603

Kommoss F, Oliva E, Bittinger F *et al* (2000) Inhibin-alpha CD99, HEA125, PLAP and chromogranin immunoreactivity in testicular neoplasms and the androgen insensitivity syndrome. *Hum Pathol* **31**: 1055–61

Meinardi MT, Gietema JA, van der Graaf WT *et al* (2000) Cardiovascular morbidity in long-term survivors of metastatic testicular cancer. *J Clin Oncol* **18**: 1725–32

Motzer R, Bosl G, Heelan R *et al* (1987) Residual mass: an indication for further therapy in patients with advanced seminoma following systemic chemotherapy. *J Clin Oncol* **5**: 1064–70

Moul JW, Foley JP, Hitchcock CL *et al* (1993) Flow cytometric and quantitative histological parameters to predict occult disease in clinical stage I non-seminomatous testicular germ cell tumors. *J Urol* **150**: 879–83

Oliver RT (2001) Testicular cancer. *Curr Opin Oncol* **13**: 191–8

Otite U, Webb JA, Oliver RT, Badenoch DF, Nargund VH (2001) Testicular microlithiasis: is it a benign condition with malignant potential? *Eur Urol* **40**: 538–42

Peterson AC, Bauman JM, Light DE, McMann LP, Costabile RA (2001) The prevalence of testicular microlithiasis in an asymptomatic population of men 18–35 years old. *J Urol* **166**: 2061–4

Pugh RCB, Cameron K (1976) *Teratoma*. Blackwell Scientific Publications, Oxford

Quinn M, Babb P, Brock A, Kirby L, Jones J (2001) *Cancer Trends in England and Wales, 1950–1999.* Office for National Statistics, London

Rapley EA, Crockford GP, Teare D *et al* (2000) Localization to Xq27 of a susceptibility gene for testicular germ-cell tumours. *Nat Genet* **24**: 197–200

Read G, Stenning SP, Cullen MH *et al* (1992) Medical Research Council prospective study of surveillance for stage I testicular teratoma. Medical Research Council Testicular Tumors Working Party. *J Clin Oncol* **10**: 1762–8

Royal College of Radiologists (2002) Evidence-based guidelines. Royal College of Radiologists, London. Available at: http://www.rcr.ac.uk/oncologytemplate.asp?PageID=209 Accessed 19 July 2002

Sharpe RM, Skakkebaek NE (1993) Are oestrogens involved in falling sperm counts and disorders of the male reproductive tract? *Lancet* **341**: 1392–5

Strohmeyer T, Peter S, Hartmann M et al (1991) Expression of the hst-1 and c-kit protooncogenes in human testicular germ cell tumors. *Cancer Res* **51**: 1811–16

Travis LB, Andersson M, Gospodarowicz M *et al* (2000) Treatment-associated leukemia following testicular cancer. *J Natl Cancer Inst* **92**: 1165–71

Key points

⌘ Testicular cancer is the commonest cancer in men aged twenty to thirty-four years of age.

⌘ Men should be made aware of testicular cancer and its presenting symptoms, especially if there is a history of maldescended testis or family history of testicular cancer.

⌘ Advanced and recurrent disease should be managed by a multidisciplinary team.

⌘ Microlithiasis may be associated with testicular cancer and may be a precursor lesion.

⌘ Routine testicular self-examination is helpful.

6

Penile cancer: an overview

Iqbal Shergill, Manit Arya, Hitendra RH Patel

Carcinoma of the penis affects one in 100 000 men each year in most developed countries. Survival is excellent if diagnosed early, but most men present up to one year after the initial lesion is noted. Unfortunately, the treatment of metastatic disease is still disappointing.

Introduction

Penile cancer is often overshadowed by other urological malignancies (prostate, bladder and testis). It does not usually present a diagnostic challenge, but its management can be difficult. Surgery has been the treatment of choice in the past, but with the advancement of chemoradiotherapy and the severe psychological and physical consequences associated with extensive surgery the emphasis has shifted to penile preservation.

Epidemiology

Penile cancer affects one in 100 000 men each year in the USA and Europe (Mobilio and Ficarra, 2001). In certain areas of Africa, Asia and South America the incidence may reach nineteen in

100 000 men each year (Hakenberg and Wirth, 1999). Penile cancer accounts for 0.4–0.6% of malignancies in the USA and Europe, but may constitute up to 10% of malignancies in African and some South American countries (Gloecklec-Ries, 1990). Men over the age of sixty years are predominantly affected (Persky, 1977). However, a significant proportion (22%) of these tumours appear in men under forty years of age (Dean, 1935).

Risk factors

Poor hygiene

Poor hygiene has commonly been associated with penile cancer. Penile cancer occurs with higher frequency in uncircumcized men with congenital phimosis, and is rare in men circumcized at birth. In India, carcinoma of the penis is almost non-existent in the neonatally circumcized Jewish population, present in prepubertal Muslims and relatively common in uncircumcized Hindus and Christians (Paymaster and Gangadharan, 1967). Adult circumcision offers little protection against penile cancer (Thomas and Small, 1963). It has been suggested that chronic penile irritation secondary to smegma accumulation or balanitis with poor hygiene are contributory factors (Mobilio and Ficarra, 2001).

Human papilloma virus

Human papilloma virus infection (types 16 and 18) has also been implicated as a risk factor for penile cancer (Picconi *et al*, 2000).

Interestingly, up to an eight-fold increase in the incidence of cervical cancer has been reported in partners of patients with carcinoma of the penis (Goldberg *et al*, 1979).

Venereal disease and trauma

Penile cancer has been documented in scarred penis after mutilating circumcision (Bissada *et al*, 1986), but the correlation is thought to be incidental. Similarly, there is no consistent relationship between penile cancer and venereal disease (Schrek and Lenowitz, 1947).

Pathology

Premalignant dermatological lesions

Balanitis xerotica obliterans (BXO), or newly termed lichen sclerosis atrophicus, is an idiopathic condition caused by abnormal collagen deposition and histiocytic infiltration (Layman and Freeman, 1944). There are reports documenting the development of penile cancer even after the excision of BXO (Dore *et al*, 1990).

Leucoplakia appears as solitary or multiple whitish lesions. Histologically, hyperkeratosis, parakeratosis and lymphocytic infiltration are seen. There is an association with squamous cell carcinoma *in situ* (Bain and Geronemus, 1989).

Virus-related dermatological lesions

Buschke–Lowenstein tumour (giant condylomata acuminata) are believed to be of viral origin, particularly human papilloma virus types 16, 18 and 31 (Smotkin, 1989). They are soft papillomatous growths and are generally considered to be non-metastatic, although they have been associated with penile carcinoma (Rhatigan *et al*, 1972).

Kaposi's sarcoma was first described in 1972 as a tumour of the reticuloendothelial system (Kaposi, 1982). It is now closely linked with acquired immune deficiency syndrome (AIDS) when it is more aggressive. Penile involvement is more common in AIDS patients who are homosexual than in those who are intravenous drug abusers or haemophiliacs (Bayne and Wise, 1988).

Carcinoma in situ

Erythroplasia of Queyrat, or Bowen's disease, is eponymous with carcinoma *in situ* of the penis and surrounding genital region. Lesions involving the glans, prepuce and shaft are called erythroplasia, while those affecting the remainder of the genitalia and perineal area are referred to as Bowen's disease. Clinically, these lesions present as erythematous plaques. Microscopically, they reveal hyperplastic cells with mitotic figures and vacuolated cytoplasm. If left untreated, carcinoma *in situ* of the penis may regress. However, up to one-third of these patients will develop invasive carcinoma (Mikhail, 1980).

Invasive carcinoma

Squamous cell carcinoma accounts for 95% of all penile cancer, with approximately 40% of patients presenting with superficial disease at diagnosis. Squamous cell carcinoma is slow to metastasize to inguinal and subsequently pelvic lymph nodes. Haematogenous spread to lungs, liver and bone occurs in <10% of patients (Puras *et al*, 1978).

Verrucous carcinoma constitutes approximately 5% of penile

cancer (Adriazola-Semino *et al*, 1990). Although the histological picture appears benign, the lesion behaves as a low-grade squamous cell carcinoma with invasion through the basement membrane occurring late in its evolution. Metastasis is extremely rare (Lopez Alcina *et al*, 1996).

Rarely, penile basal cell carcinoma may occur.

Presentation

Presenting symptoms and signs are shown in *Table 6.1*.

The majority of lesions are not painful, which may explain why up to 50% of patients delay a medical opinion for at least one year from the time of initial awareness of the lesion (Dean, 1935). At presentation approximately 50% of patients have palpable inguinal nodes, but these usually represent an inflammatory response rather than metastasis.

Table 6.1: Presenting symptoms and signs of penile cancer

- Epithelial thickening on glans or inner prepuce
- Ulcerative or exophytic growth
- Penile discharge or dysuria
- Bleeding
- Palpable inguinal nodes

The exposure to smegma may explain the observed tumour distribution:

- glans (48%)
- prepuce (21%)
- both glans and prepuce (9%)
- coronal sulcus (6%)
- shaft (<2%)
- a combination in 14% (Sufrin and Huben, 1991).

Diagnosis

Diagnosis is confirmed by an incisional biopsy. A pelvic magnetic resonance imaging (MRI) scan is the investigation of choice to assess the extent of local invasion. If locally advanced, further clinical staging should include a computed tomography (CT) scan of the abdomen, chest X-ray and isotope bone scan. Less than 10% of patients present with metastasis. In the absence of osseous metastasis, hypercalcaemia is seen in up to 20% of cases, correlating with the volume of the disease (Sklaroff and Yagoda, 1982).

Staging

The most commonly used staging system is the tumour, node, metastasis (TNM) classification of the American Joint Committee on Cancer (1997), as shown in *Table 6.2* (and also described in *Chapter 2*).

Table 6.2: Tumour, node, metastasis (TNM) classification of penile cancer

Primary tumour (T)	TX	Primary tumour cannot be assessed
	T0	No evidence of primary tumour
	Tis	Carcinoma in situ
	Ta	Non-invasive verrucous carcinoma
	T1	Tumour invades subepithelial connective tissue
	T2	Tumour invades corpus spongiosum or cavernosum
	T3	Tumour invades urethra or prostate
	T4	Tumour invades other adjacent structures
Regional lymph nodes (N)	NX	Regional lymph nodes cannot be assessed
	N0	No regional lymph node metastases
	N1	Metastasis in a single superficial inguinal lymph node
	N2	Metastasis in multiple or bilateral superficial inguinal lymph nodes
	N3	Metastasis in deep inguinal or pelvic lymph node(s), unilateral or bilateral
Distant metastasis (M)	MX	Distant metastasis cannot be assessed
	M0	No distant metastasis
	M1	Distant metastasis

From American Joint Committee on Cancer (1997)

Treatment

Treatment options for carcinoma *in situ*, verrucous carcinoma and the primary lesion in squamous carcinoma are shown in *Table 6.3* (Hakenberg and Wirth, 1999; Agrawal *et al*, 2000).

Table 6.3: Treatment options for localized penile cancer

Carcinoma *in situ*	Laser ablation	
	Local excision	
	Topical chemotherapy (5-fluorouracil)	
	External beam radiotherapy	
Verrucous carcinoma	Partial penectomy	
	Total penectomy	
Squamous cell carcinoma	T1/T2 tumours*	Partial penectomy
		Laser ablation
		Yttrium aluminium garnet or carbon dioxide laser
	T3 Total penectomy†	
	T4 Emasculation	

*Recently, more conservative surgery with maximum preservation of penile length and function has been increasingly used for the management for T1 tumours confined to the glans (Mobilio and Ficarra, 2001). These penile-sparing treatments result in less emotional impact than radical surgery, but have been shown by some studies to have a high rate of local recurrence ranging from 32–50% (Mobilio and Ficarra, 2001).

†External beam radiotherapy for T3 neoplasms has been reported to have a high risk of recurrence (Fossa *et al*, 1987).

Other penile tumours

Although more than 95% of cases of penile cancer are squamous cell carcinomas, cases of basal cell carcinoma, Paget's disease and melanoma have been reported. The increase in human immunodeficiency virus infection has lead to an increased incidence of Kaposi's sarcoma; this tumour is highly radiosensitive.

Palpable nodes

Inguinal lymph nodes represent the first site of distant dissemination of penile carcinoma. Their involvement and the manner in which they are managed are the most important determinants of patient survival in penile cancer.

Approximately 50% of patients will have palpable lymph nodes at presentation. Of this group only 15–45% will actually have metastatic tumour involvement, while the remainder will have lymphadenopathy caused by inflammation of the penis. A four to five-week course of antibiotics will usually cause a complete regression of lymphadenopathy in the latter group.

If lymphadenopathy persists after antibiotic treatment, bilateral lymphadenectomy is advised, provided chest X-ray and abdominopelvic CT or MRI scans are normal, as this may be curative. If the patient is not fit for this procedure, radiotherapy to the nodes is an alternative.

If nodes are fixed to the superficial and deep layers, inguinal lymphadenectomy is not advised as surgical excision may be difficult and incomplete, resulting in a high rate of morbidity. These patients should be treated with chemotherapy and, if there is a response, lymphadenectomy may be performed.

Non-palpable nodes

The most controversial issue is that of inguinal lymphadenectomy in patients with clinically negative nodes. Up to 20% of these patients have nodal micrometastasis and would benefit from early lymph node dissection (Mobilio and Ficarra, 2001). However, prophylactic lymph node dissection in the remaining 80% renders them liable to significant complications, including mortality in up to 3%, skin necrosis in up to 60% and lower limb lymphoedema in up to 25% of patients (Hakenberg and Wirth, 1999). Thus in patients with clinically negative nodes, the decision of prophylactic lymph node dissection is based on the pathological stage and grade of the primary tumour.

Patients with well-differentiated pT1 tumours and clinically impalpable nodes have a low risk of micrometastatic node involvement and may be managed by surveillance without lymphadenectomy. Patients with poorly differentiated and pT2–4 neoplasms have nodal micrometastases in up to 83% of cases, thus bilateral inguinal lymphadenectomy is recommended (Bouchot *et al*, 1997).

Metastatic disease

Success rates for metastatic disease are poor. Most treatment protocols rely on chemotherapeutic agents such as bleomycin, cisplatin and methotrexate. This may result in a 60% response rate, although this is usually short-lived, with a mean duration of response being six months (Hakenberg and Wirth, 1999).

Prognosis

The five-year survival values are shown in *Table 6.4*.

Table 6.4: Five-year survival figures for penile cancer	
Stage at diagnosis	**5-year survival**
Node-negative squamous cell carcinoma	65–90%
Inguinal node metastases	30–50%
Iliac node metastases	<20%
Soft tissue or bony metastases	0%

From Algaba *et al* (2000)

Follow up

Specialist centres follow these patients according to the grade and stage of the tumour, in a multidisciplinary setting. Follow up should include a physical examination, which in turn will dictate the need to perform an abdominal CT scan, inguinal MRI or a chest X-ray.

Conclusions

A better understanding of progression of penile carcinoma has led to improved survival in organ-confined disease and preservation of the penis. Unfortunately, similar results have not been achieved in metastatic disease. It is expected that with advancement in chemoradiotherapy, improved survival for advanced disease will be achieved.

References

Adriazola-Semino M, Aparicio R, Lozano JL, Tejeda E, Amo Garcia A, Romero F (1990) Verrucous carcinoma of the penis. Presentation of 3 new cases. [Spanish] *Actas Urol Esp* **14**(6): 435–6

Agrawal A, Pai D, Ananthakrishnan N, Smile SR, Ratnakar C (2000) The histological extent of the local spread of carcinoma of the penis and its therapeutic implications. *Br J Urol Int* **85**(3): 299–301

Algaba F, Horenblas S, Pizzocaro G *et al* (2000) *Guidelines on Penile Cancer*. Presented at the European Association of Urology, Brussels, 11–15 April

American Joint Committee on Cancer (1997) *AJCC Cancer Staging Manual*. 5th edn. Lippencott Raven Publishers, Philadelphia PA

Bain L, Geronemus R (1989) The association of lichen planus of the penis with squamous cell carcinoma *in situ* and with verrucous squamous carcinoma. *J Dermatol Surg Oncol* **15**(4): 413–17

Bayne D, Wise GJ (1988) Kaposi sarcoma of penis and genitalia: a disease of our times. *Urology* **31**(1): 22–5

Bissada NK, Morcos RR, el-Senoussi M (1986) Post-circumcision carcinoma of the penis. I. Clinical aspects. *J Urol* **135**(2): 283–5

Bouchot O, Boullanger P, Buzelin JM (1997) Inguinal lymphadenctomy in cancer of the penis: surgical techniques and indications. [French]. *Prog Urol* **7**: 665–73

Dean AL (1935) Epithelioma of the penis. *J Urol* **33**: 252

Dore B, Irani J, Aubert J (1990) Carcinoma of the penis in lichen sclerosus atrophicus. A case report. *Eur Urol* **18**(2): 153–5

Fossa SD, Hall KS, Johannessen NB, Urnes T, Kaalhus O (1987) Cancer of the penis. Experience at the Norwegian Radium Hospital 1974–1985. *Eur Urol* **13**(6): 372–7

Gloecklec-Ries LA (1990) *Cancer Statistics Review 1973–1987*. Hankey BF, Edwards BF, eds. NIH Pub No 90–2789. National Cancer Institute, NIH, Bethesda

Goldberg HM, Pell-Ilderton R, Daw E, Saleh N (1979) Concurrent squamous cell carcinoma of the cervix and penis in a married couple. *Br J Obstet Gynaecol* **86**(7): 585–6

Hakenberg OW, Wirth MP (1999) Issues in the treatment of penile carcinoma. A short review. *Urol Int* **62**(4): 229–33

Kaposi M (1982) Idiopathic multiple pigmented sarcoma of skin. [Reproduced from *Arch Derm Syphil* **4**: 265, 1892] *Cancer* **32**: 342

Layman CW, Freeman C (1944) Relationship between BXO to lichen sclerosis et atrophicus. *Arch Dermatol Syph* **49**: 57

Lopez Alcina E, Rodrigo Aliaga M, Martinez Samiento M *et al* (1996) Verrucous carcinoma of the penis. *Acta Urol Esp* **20**: 560–3

Mikhail GR (1980) Cancers, precancers, and pseudocancers on the male genitalia. A review of clinical appearances, histopathology and management. *J Dermatol Surg Oncol* **6**(12): 1027–35

Mobilio G, Ficarra V (2001) Genital treatment of penile carcinoma. *Curr Opin Urol* **11**(3): 299–304

Paymaster JC, Gangadharan P (1967) Cancer of the penis in India. *J Urol* **97**(1): 110–13

Persky L (1977) Epidemiology of carcinoma of penis. *Rec Results Cancer Research* **60**: 97–109

Picconi MA, Eijan AM, Distefano AL *et al* (2000) A human papillomavirus DNA in penile carcinomas in Argentina: analysis of primary tumors and lymph nodes. *J Med Virol* **61**(1): 65–9

Puras A, Gonzales-Flores B, Furtuno B (1978) Treatment of carcinoma of penis. *Proc Kimborough Urol Semin* **12**: 143

Rhatigan RM, Jimenez S, Chopskie EJ (1972) Condyloma accuminata and carcinoma of penis. *South Med J* **65**: 423

Schrek R, Lenowitz H (1947) Etiologic factors in carcinoma of penis. *Cancer Res* **7**: 180

Sklaroff RB, Yagoda A (1982) Penile cancer: natural history and therapy. In: Spiers ASD, ed. *Chemotherapy and Urological Malignancy*. Springer-Verlag, London: 111–19

Smotkin D (1989) Virology of human papillomavirus. *Clin Obstet Gynecol* **32**(1): 117–26

Sufrin G, Huben R (1991) Benign and malignant lesions of penis. In: Gillenwater JY, ed. *Adult and Paediatric Urology*. 2nd edn. Chicago Year Book Medical Publishers, St Louis: 1643

Thomas JA, Small CS (1963) Carcinoma of the penis in Southern India. *J Urol* **100**(4): 520–6

Key points

✤ Carcinoma of the penis presents as an obvious lesion; however, 50% of patients may delay seeking medical opinion up to one year from the time of initial awareness.

✤ Neonatal circumcision and good hygiene afford protection against penile cancer.

✤ Diagnosis has to be confirmed by biopsy.

✤ Surgery offers the best chance of cure in localized penile carcinoma.

✤ The rise in incidence of the human immunodeficiency virus has resulted in increased cases of Kaposi's sarcoma, especially in homosexual men.

✤ Chemoradiation is increasingly being used to control localized disease in order to preserve organ function.

✤ The advancement in chemoradiation therapies is expected to result in better prognosis for patients with carcinoma of the penis.

7

Paediatric genitourinary malignances

Venita Patel

Paediatric genitourinary tumours are rarely seen in clinical practice. However, clinicians must be aware of these cancers, as early treatment gives a better prognosis.

Introduction

Most people will not come across paediatric genitourinary tumours, although it is important to remember them when involved with any aspect of child health. Early detection and prompt therapy have the potential to reduce mortality. One must be alert for possible presenting signs and symptoms, especially in patients with congenital or familial conditions associated with an increased risk of cancer.

The main tumours to be aware of include:

- Wilms' tumour (nephroblastoma)
- neuroblastoma
- rhabdomyosarcoma
- testicular cancer.

The aim of this chapter is to provide a summary of the main uro-oncological cancers affecting children, and a brief outline of their diagnosis and management.

Wilms' tumour (nephroblastoma)

Epidemiology

The most common neoplasm of the urinary tract in children is Wilms' tumour, which accounts for 8% of all paediatric solid tumours. The mean age of presentation is at three years, and both sexes are equally affected (Breslow *et al*, 1993). The tumour is 50% more prevalent in AfroCaribbean populations (Breslow *et al*, 1994).

Aetiology/pathology

Various genes on chromosome 11 have been associated with Wilms' tumour, and also with the predisposing congenital syndromes — Beckwith–Wiedemann, Denys–Drash and WAGR (Haiken and Miller, 1971; Pendergrass, 1976; Narahara *et al*, 1984; Petruzzi and Green, 1997). The tumour is a solitary growth in any part of the kidney, usually encapsulated and distorting the normal anatomy. The classic pathology is a nephroblastoma with three types of cells, which occurs in 90% of cases and has a good prognosis; the remaining 10% have unfavourable histology, with rhabdoid, clear cell and anaplastic features (Beckwith, 1983).

Diagnosis

The typical presentation of Wilms' tumour is of a painless abdominal mass in a generally well child, which is smooth and rarely crosses the midline. Bleeding into the tumour can cause pain, and tumour rupture secondary to trauma can present as an acute abdomen. Haematuria is seen in 10–25% of cases, with 63% having hypertension (Ramsey *et al*, 1977).

Abdominal ultrasound can usually confirm the diagnosis, and is used to assess extension into vessels, particularly as 20% invade the renal vein. Up to 15% of patients will have metastatic disease at primary diagnosis (D'Angio *et al*, 1989).

Treatment

Management consists of surgery with chemotherapy, and radiotherapy is also used depending on tumour stage and pathology (D'Angio *et al*, 1989). Computed tomography (CT) and magnetic resonance imaging (MRI) are used to evaluate the size of the tumour, the precise anatomy and the presence of bilateral disease; however, 7% of these are missed on imaging, and surgery therefore includes exploration of the other kidney (Ritchey *et al*, 1995).

Neoadjuvant chemotherapy drugs are used (vincristine, actinomycin D and doxorubicin). In bilateral disease, biopsies are initially taken, followed by chemotherapy, to preserve any healthy renal tissue.

Prognosis

In classical Wilms' tumour, the four-year survival rate ranges from 60% for stage IV to 90% for stage I/II (D'Angio *et al*, 1989). With unfavourable histology, the rates are:

- 20% for rhabdoid
- 60% for anaplastic
- 60–70% for clear cell.

Up to half of all relapses are, however, still curable, particularly in children with abdominal relapse who have not had previous radiation. Metastatic disease worsens the overall prognosis.

Neuroblastoma

Neuroblastoma is mentioned because it is an important differential diagnosis when Wilms' tumour is suspected (see above). Neuroblastoma arises from neural crest cells, and can occur in sites along the sympathetic chain from head to pelvis. Over half are abdominal (two-thirds are adrenal), and the mass is firm, irregular and extends beyond the midline. It is unusual as it may also regress spontaneously in young infants, or differentiate to benign tumours (Brodeur *et al*, 1993).

Epidemiology

Neuroblastoma is the second most common solid tumour of childhood, affecting the sexes almost equally. Fifty percent occur in children under two years old, and 75% are diagnosed before the age of four years (Miller *et al*, 1968). It is important to note that the incidence may be increasing, as shown in a recent study from the north of England (Cotterill *et al*, 2001).

Aetiology/pathology

The clinical behaviour of neuroblastoma is variable and may represent a multitude of genetic aberrations leading to the different phenotypes (Bown, 2001). These tumours display a spectrum of histological maturation and differentiation.

Diagnosis

Most children present with an abdominal mass and associated symptoms of catecholamine secretion (sweating, pallor, palpitations, weight loss and headaches). Over the age of two years, symptoms of metastatic disease may also present with malaise, bone pain and hepatomegaly.

Urinary catecholamines are raised, and anaemia is common at presentation. Studies to help confirm diagnosis include CT scanning, with biopsy. Metastatic disease is detected by bone scan, bone marrow sampling and MIBG (meta-iodo-benzyl-guanidine) scan.

Treatment

Poor prognostic factors, including increasing age and tumour stage, determine the treatment protocols. Surgery is the mainstay, with radiotherapy to the bed of the excision for localized disease. Large but localized masses can be treated with neoadjuvant radiotherapy before surgical excision. If the disease is metastatic, chemotherapy is used as the primary treatment.

Prognosis

Low-risk patients can be cured with surgery alone, and have a 95% five-year survival.

Intermediate-risk patients have favourable histological phenotype and molecular amplification (MYCN oncogene; Bown, 2001). These patients are treated by chemotherapy and surgery, with survival ranging from 55–90% at five years.

The remaining patients make up the high-risk group; they have multimodal treatment, with poor five-year survival (20%; Katzenstein and Cohn, 1998).

Rhabdomyosarcoma

Epidemiology

Rhabdomyosarcoma is a rare soft-tissue sarcoma. The genitourinary tract accounts for 10–15% of all cases of rhabdomyosarcoma (Maurer et al, 1988). It has two peak ages of incidence: <2 years (affecting the neck, head, vagina, bladder and prostate) and fifteen to nineteen years (affecting the genitourinary tract, especially the testes/paratestes) (La Quaglia *et al*, 1994). There is an increased incidence in males to females (3:1) (deVries, 1995).

Aetiology/pathology

Rhabdomyosarcoma arises from embryonic (undifferentiated) mesenchymal tissue, and has several histological subtypes (Newton *et al*, 1988):

- embryonal (including botyroid)
- alveolar
- pleomorphic.

Most genitourinary tumours are embryonal, and histology shows features of mature skeletal muscle with cross-striations and rhabdomyoblasts. Dissemination is by local invasion in most cases, by lymphatic spread in 18%, and by distant metastases to lung/bone in 10%.

Diagnosis

Clinical presentation depends on tumour location, and is commonly a large palpable mass in the abdomen, with pain. Other symptoms include urgency and frequency, recurrent urinary tract infections and rarely haematuria, which tend to be abdominal mass pressure effects. In girls, there may be a protruding grape-like vaginal mass (botyroid tumour).

Investigation involves a chest X-ray, ultrasound of the pelvis and urinary tract, and CT or MRI to determine spread. Bone marrow examination and routine blood tests are required, as is histological assessment via biopsy.

Treatment

Current management begins with neoadjuvant combination chemotherapy (vincristine, actinomycin D, cyclophosphamide) for eight weeks before surgery or radiotherapy is contemplated (Pappo *et al*, 1997).

Prognosis

In children with early-stage disease, the five-year survival rate is 75–81%, with over half of the patients with bladder/prostate involvement retaining their bladders (Hays *et al*, 1995). The outlook for metastatic disease is poor at around 20%, despite radiation to the affected sites (Pappo *et al*, 1997).

Testicular cancer

Testicular tumours account for 2% of all paediatric solid tumours. The peak incidence is in two-year-olds, with two-thirds being germ cell tumours and the rest being benign. This cancer is discussed in more detail in *Chapter 5*.

Conclusions

Paediatric genitourinary malignancies are rarely seen across clinical practice. Indeed, highly specialized centres deal with their management. Advances in our knowledge of these tumours are being made in both the scientific and clinical fields. However, survival has also improved significantly by effective multidisciplinary care. Thus, when presented with a mass in a child, a background awareness of these cancers is important for early detection.

References

Beckwith JB (1983) Wilms' tumor and other renal tumors of childhood: a selective review from the National Wilms' Tumor Study Pathology Center. *Hum Pathol* **14**: 481–92

Bown N (2001) Neuroblastoma tumour genetics: clinical and biological aspects. *J Clin Pathol* **54**: 897–910

Breslow NE, Olshan A, Beckwith JB, Green DM (1993) Epidemiology of Wilms' tumor. *Med Pediatr Oncol* **21**: 172–81

Breslow NE, Olshan A, Beckwith JB *et al* (1994) Ethnic variation in the incidence, diagnosis, prognosis and follow up of children with Wilms' tumor. *J Natl Cancer Inst* **86**: 49–51

Brodeur GM, Pritchard J, Berthold F *et al* (1993) Revisions of the international criteria for neuroblastoma diagnosis, staging and response to treatment. *J Clin Oncol* **11**: 1466–77

Cotterill SJ, Parker L, More L, Craft AW (2001) Neuroblastoma: changing incidence and survival in young people aged 0–24 years. A report from the north of England young persons' malignant disease registry. *Med Ped Oncol* **36**: 231–4

D'Angio GJ, Breslow NB, Beckwith JB et al (1989) Treatment of Wilms' tumor: results of the third national Wilms' tumor study. *Cancer* **64**: 349–60

Haiken BN, Miller DR (1971) Simultaneous occurrence of congenital aniridia, haematoma and Wilms' tumor. *J Paediatr* **78**: 497–502

Hays DM, Raney RB, Wharam MD *et al* (1995) Children with vesical rhabdomyosarcoma treated by partial cystectomy with neoadjuvant chemotherapy, with or without radiotherapy: a report from the intergroup rhabdomyosarcoma study committee. *J Pediatr Hematol Oncol* **17**: 46–52

Katzenstein HM, Cohn SL (1998) Advances in the diagnosis and treatment of neuroblastoma. *Curr Opin Oncol* **10**: 43–51

La Quaglia M, Heller G, Ghavami F *et al* (1994) The effect of age at diagnosis on outcome in rhabdomyosarcoma. *Cancer* **73**: 109–117

Maurer HM, Beltangady M, Geham EA et al (1988) The intergroup rhabdomyosarcoma study I: a final report. *Cancer* **61**: 209–20

Miller RW, Fraumeni JF, Hill JA (1968) Neuroblastoma: epidemiologic approach to its origin. *Am J Dis Child* **115**: 253–61

Narahara K, Kikkawa S, Kimira S *et al* (1984) Regional mapping of catalase and Wilms' tumor: aniridia, genitourinary abnormalities and mental retardation triad loci to the chromosome segment 11p1305 p1306. *Hum Genet* **66**: 181–5

Newton W, Soule EH, Hamoude A *et al* (1988) Histopathology of childhood sarcomas, intergroup rhabdomyosarcoma studies I and II: clinicopathologic classification. *J Clin Oncol* **6**: 67–75

Pappo AS, Shapiro DN, Crist WM (1997) Rhabdomyosarcoma: biology and treatment. *Pediatr Clin North Am* **44**: 953–72

Petruzzi MJ, Green DM (1997) Wilms' tumor. *Pediatr Clin North Am* **44**: 939–52

Pendergrass TW (1976) Congenital anomalies in children with Wilms' tumor. *Cancer* **37**: 3–8

Ramsey NK, Dehner LP, Cowcia PF *et al* (1977) Acute hemorrhage into Wilms' tumor: a cause of rapidly developing abdominal mass with hypertension, anemia and fever. *J Pediatr* **91**: 763–5

Ritchey ML, Green DM, Breslow NB *et al* (1995) Accuracy of current imaging modalities in the diagnosis of synchronous bilateral Wilms' tumor. A report from the national Wilms' tumor study group. *Cancer* **75**: 600–4

deVries JD (1995) Paratesticular rhabdomyosarcoma. *World J Urol* **13**: 219–25

Key points

❈ Paediatric genitourinary tumours are rarely seen in clinical practice.

❈ The most common neoplasm of the urinary tract in children is Wilms' tumour, which accounts for 8% of all paediatric solid tumours.

❈ An important differential diagnosis is neuroblastoma.

❈ Rhabdomyosarcoma is a rare soft-tissue sarcoma, accounting for 10–15% of all solid tumours in childhood.

❈ A background awareness of these cancers is important for early detection, thus giving a better prognosis.

8

New horizons in urological oncology

Ahsan Haq and Hitendra RH Patel

Advances in DNA and chromosomal analysis, imaging and microchip technology, and the publication of the DNA sequence of the entire genome create an unparalleled opportunity for discovery. This chapter outlines recent findings and developments in the prevention, detection and treatment of urological tumours.

Introduction

The recent advances in the biological sciences, technology and the deciphering of the human genome have brought with them the prospect of understanding urological tumours on a previously unimaginable level. The three areas in urological tumour therapy that need to be enhanced are:

- prevention
- early diagnosis of localized disease, with available effective therapy and minimal toxicity or impact on quality of life
- effective treatment of advanced disease (this will remain necessary for many years to come until improved molecular understanding of the causes of tumour development, growth and progression are unravelled).

Dietary influences on prostate cancer

Autopsy series demonstrate that the incidence of latent prostate cancer is approximately equal in Asian and American men (Breslow *et al*, 1997). African-Americans have the highest incidence of clinical prostate cancer, which is up to thirty times greater than that in Japanese men, and 120 times greater than that observed in Chinese men (Parkin *et al*, 1992). Japanese migrants to the USA experience an increase in incidence to approximately half the indigenous population within one or two generations (Wang *et al*, 1995). This fast epidemiological change and international comparisons in diet demonstrate that dietary differences such as fat and soy consumption may be partly responsible for the phenomenon.

Fat consumption as a dietary factor relating to carcinoma risk has received much recent attention. That dietary fat reduction may help prevent prostate cancer is supported by numerous case-control studies reported over the past several decades (Heshmat *et al*, 1985; Kolonel *et al*, 1988). It is difficult to draw conclusions from these studies, however, because of the greater potential for recall bias and confounding variables. Therefore, large-scale prospective studies were performed to shed a light on this issue (Schuurman *et al*, 1999; Hanash *et al*, 2000). These prospective studies have arrived at differing conclusions from previous studies, and have not shown a significant impact on prostate cancer by reducing dietary fat. Clinicians should be careful not to suggest such a benefit until more research provides a better picture of the situation.

Fat reduction, together with soy products or other plant oestrogen foods, may have a symbiotic relationship. Numerous healthy lifestyle changes practised at one time (healthy diet, attainment of normal weight, soy consumption) may hold some promise in the area of cancer prevention. In the meantime, any healthy lifestyle or dietary changes should be encouraged as they reduce the risk of cardiovascular disease, which is still the number one cause of mortality and is also an important cause of morbidity and mortality in cancer patients.

Genetic basis of renal cell carcinoma

Advances in DNA and chromosomal analysis, imaging and microchip technology, and the publication of the DNA sequence of the entire genome create an unparalleled opportunity for discovery. In the past, cytogenetic research relied upon classic G-banding of chromosomes, a notoriously challenging endeavour with solid tumour karyotypes. Spectral karyotyping applied to renal cell carcinomas (RCCs) enables the simultaneous visualization of all chromosomes in unique colours (Philips *et al*, 2001).

Spectral karyotyping is invaluable in identifying chromosomal breakpoints that are too complex or subtle for traditional techniques, and in refining the search for new genes. Comparative genomic hybridization enables the assessment of which chromosomal regions are gained or lost in tumours (Yang *et al*, 2000).

A combination of spectral karyotyping and comparative genomic hybridization data, in an Internet-accessible database (see http://www.ncbi.nlm.nih.gov/sky/skyweb.cgi), has tremendous diagnostic and prognostic potential. Microarrays of cDNAs enable the simultaneous assessment of thousands of genes, or in the case of tissue microarrays, hundreds of tumour samples (Moch *et al*, 1999). Now researchers have the tools to understand the carcinoma cell in real time: the simultaneous interaction and clustering of gene expression patterns to provide a cancer cell with a growth advantage.

There is no medical cure for patients with metastatic RCC, and only patients with organ-confined disease who undergo radical nephrectomy will experience long-term survival. Of all the therapies for the treatment of metastatic RCC, the Food and Drug Administration in the USA currently approves only interleukin-2 (IL-2)-based immunotherapy; thus better therapies are required for the vast majority of patients.

Molecular targeting-based therapy has the attraction of targeting the cancer cell for what causes it, ie. a dysregulation of genes important to renal homeostasis. It is too early to say whether replacement of the function of the missing Von Hippel Lindau tumour-suppressor gene will be sufficient to arrest tumour growth, as the recognized tumour-suppressor genes are among a number of genes that have become dysregulated by the time tumours reach clinical significance.

An alternative approach would be the design of therapies to make RCCs more susceptible to conventional treatments such as chemotherapy or radiation, against which RCCs are notoriously refractory. Preliminary molecular targeting studies suggest that such strategies may well enhance immune-mediated tumour cell killing (Schendel *et al*, 2000) and sensitivity to alkylating agents.

Allogenic stem cell transplantation is a potent form of immunotherapy capable of delivering potentially curative immune-mediated anti-tumour effects against a number of different haematological malignancies. Knowledge of RCCs' unusual susceptibility to immune attack has led to the hypothesis that tumour rejection, mediated through immunocompetent donor T-cells, might be generated against this solid tumour following the transplantation of an allogenic immune system. Clinical trials are early and ongoing, but the recent observation of metastatic disease regression following non-myeloablative stem cell transplantation has identified RCC as being susceptible to graft *vs* tumour effect (Childs *et al*, 2000). Disease responses following such therapy have ranged from partial to complete, and have been seen even in patients who have failed conventional cytokine-based treatment.

Laparoscopic surgery in urological pelvic cancer

Laparoscopic surgery has become more widely used in urological practice, initially for upper and more recently for the lower urinary tract. Laparoscopy for nephrectomy was the first and finest example of the application and its advantages in urological practice. Over the past ten years, with the improvements in instrumentation and the experience of surgeons, the applications of laparoscopy have broadened. It is now possible to perform major pelvic procedures laparoscopically with a combination of resection and urinary tract reconstruction.

Guilloneau and Vallencien (2000) described the 'Montsouris technique' of radical prostatectomy. The specific features of the operative technique include the transperitoneal approach, visual control, dissection using forceps (bipolar coagulation) and scissors (unipolar cutting current). The conversion rate for the first forty patients was 10%, and 0% for the last 160 patients. The mean operating time was down to 206 minutes for the last 140 patients, and in this group the transfusion rate was only 1.4%. The postoperative course in these patients also compares favourably with the open approach with respect to catheterization and thromboembolic, gastrointestinal and urinary morbidity.

The functional results are encouraging, with rapid recovery of continence in 84% of patients at 1 month (Abbou *et al*, 2000). The published results regarding sexual potency, however, are too early to permit meaningful analysis. There is no doubt that with improvement in the quality of vision at the surgical site, associated with improved operator experience, a significant improvement should be seen in neurovascular pedicle preservation, allowing recovery of spontaneous erections. Laparoscopic cystectomy with cutaneous urinary diversion by ileal conduit has also been reported (Gill *et al*, 2000), and larger series are awaited.

In the not too distant future, the amalgamation of laparoscopic techniques and robotics/computer assistance will further expand and enhance the indications for laparoscopic surgery in urological oncology.

Gene therapy for prostate cancer

Molecular-based novel therapeutic agents are needed to address the problem of locally recurrent, or metastatic, advanced hormone-refractory prostate cancer. Recent basic science advances in mechanisms of gene expression, vector delivery and targeting have enabled clinically relevant gene therapy to the prostate and distant sites to be feasible in the future.

A number of different approaches in gene therapy have been

explored to deliver the therapeutic effect (Steiner and Gingrich, 2000). These approaches include correcting aberrant gene expression, exploiting apoptotic cell pathways, introducing toxic or lytic suicide genes, targeting unique and critical cellular function, enhancing the immune system anti-tumour response and finally, a combination of different modalities of treatment.

The vast majority of clinical trial work done in gene therapy for prostate cancer has been focused around toxic 'suicidal' or immune-boosting therapies. These therapies often involve an adenovirus as a vector to deliver various chosen target genes (Collis *et al*, 2003).

The adenovirus has become the predominant vector in cancer gene therapy. They are non-enveloped, double-stranded, linear DNA viruses that cause benign respiratory tract infections in humans. The factors that make adenovirus a good choice for gene therapy include its stability, broad infectivity of dividing and non-dividing cells, high levels of transgene expression and lack of integration into the host chromosome (Collis *et al*, 2003).

If adenovirus gene therapy is to become a reality for the treatment of prostate cancer, there must be an improvement in DNA transfer efficiency to cells (especially at metastatic sites) and an augmentation of the levels of target gene expression and an overcoming of the immune response so that these genes can be expressed for a prolonged period. An ideal adenoviral vector system should target tumour neovascularization and the stroma as well as the cancerous prostate epithelium, and evade the immune surveillance system. Ongoing research into gene therapy for prostate cancer involves tissue-specific promoters, transgene exploration, vector design and delivery and selective vector targeting.

Can biological markers replace cystoscopy?

Cystoscopy is currently considered the gold standard for the detection and follow up of bladder carcinoma. It is not, however, without its complications; urinary tract infection in up to 10% of patients, urethral damage, and small areas of carcinoma *in situ* that may be missed. The role of urine cytology in the detection and follow up of patients is still not entirely clear (it does have a role in high-grade lesions and carcinoma *in situ*).

New laboratory and rapid assays are available that may circumvent the low sensitivity and poor reproducibility of urine cytology. The methods that have tested extensively are the nuclear matrix protein (NMP22) assay, the bladder tumour antigen (BTA) stat assay, and the BTA TRAK enzyme-linked immunosorbent assay. These outperform cytology in the detection of low-grade lesions; however, the specificity of these assays lags behind that of cytology. The data from retrospective analyses are at present insufficient to justify clinical integration, and the replacement of cystoscopy by these novel assays remains to be proven (Van der Poel and Debruyne, 2001).

References

Abbou CC, Salomon L, Hoznek A *et al* (2000) Laparoscopic radical prostatectomy: preliminary results. *Urology* **55**: 630–4

Breslow N, Chan CE, Dhom G *et al* (1997) Latent carcinoma of the prostate at autopsy in seven areas. *Int J Cancer* **20**: 680–8

Childs R, Chernoff A, Contentin N *et al* (2000) Regression of metastatic renal cell carcinoma after nonmyeloablative allogenic peripheral-blood-stem-cell transplantation. *N Engl J Med* **343**: 750–8

Collis SJ, Khater K, DeWeese TL (2003) Novel therapeutic strategies in prostate cancer management using gene therapy in combination with radiation therapy. *World J Urol* **21**(4): 275–89

Gill IS, Fergany A, Klein EA *et al* (2000) Laparoscopic radical cystoprostatectomy with ileal conduit performed completely intracorporeally: the initial two cases. *Urology* **56**: 26–9

Guilloneau B, Vallencien G (2000) Laparoscopic radical prostatectomy: the Montsouris technique. *J Urol* **163**: 1643–9

Hanash KA, Al-Othaimeen A, Kattan S *et al* (2000) Prostatic carcinoma: a nutritional disease? Conflicting data from the kingdom of Saudi Arabia. *J Urol* **164**: 1570–2

Heshmat MY, Kaul L, Kovi J *et al* (1985) Nutrition and prostate cancer: a case control study. *Prostate* **5**: 7–17

Kolonel LN, Yoshizawa CN, Hankin JH (1988) Diet and prostate cancer: a case control study in Hawaii. *Am J Epidemiol* **127**: 999–1012

Moch H, Schraml P, Bubendorf L *et al* (1999) High-throughput tissue microarray analysis to evaluate genes uncovered by cDNA microarray screening in renal cell carcinoma. *Am J Pathol* **154**: 981–6

Parkin DM, Muir CS, Whelan S *et al* (1992) *Cancer Incidence in Five Continents*. Vol. VI. IARC Scientific Publication, Lyon: 120

Philips JL, Ghadimi BM, Wangsa D *et al* (2001) Molecular cytogenetic characterization of early and late renal cell carcinomas in Von Hippel Lindau disease. *Genes Chromosomes Cancer* **31**: 1–9

Schendel DJ, Falk CS, Nossner E *et al* (2000) Gene transfer of human interferon gamma complementary DNA into a renal cell carcinoma line enhances MHC-restricted cytotoxic T-lymphocyte recognition but suppresses non-MHC restricted effector cell activity. *Gene Ther* **7**: 950–9

Schuurman AG, van den Brandt PA, Dorant E *et al* (1999) Association of energy and fat intake with prostate carcinoma risk: results from the Netherlands Cohort Study. *Cancer* **86**: 1019–27

Steiner MS, Gingrich JR (2000) Gene therapy for prostate cancer: where are we now? *J Urol* **164**: 1121–36

Van der Poel H, Debruyne FMJ (2001) Can biological markers replace cystoscopy? An update. *Curr Op Urol* **11**: 503–9

Wang Y, Corr JG, Thaler HT *et al* (1995) Decreased growth of established human prostate LNCaP tumours in nude mice fed a low fat diet. *J Natl Cancer Inst* **87**: 1456–62

Yang ZQ, Yoshida MA, Fukuda Y *et al* (2000) Molecular cytogenetic analysis of 17 renal cancer cell lines: increased copy number at 5q31-33 in cell lines from nonpapillary carcinomas. *Jpn J Cancer Res* **91**: 156–63

Key points

⌘ The recent advances in the biological sciences, technology and the deciphering of the human genome have brought with them the prospect of understanding urological tumours on a previously unimaginable level.

⌘ Spectral karyotyping and comparative genomic hybridization data enable researchers to understand the carcinoma cell in real time: the simultaneous interaction and clustering of gene expression patterns to provide a cancer cell with a growth advantage.

⌘ Molecular targeting-based therapy has the attraction of targeting the renal cancer cell for what causes it, ie. a dysregulation of genes important to renal homeostasis.

⌘ In the not too distant future, the amalgamation of laparoscopic techniques and robotics/computer assistance will further expand and enhance the indications for laparoscopic surgery in urological oncology.

⌘ Molecular-based novel therapeutic agents are needed to address the problem of locally recurrent, or metastatic, advanced hormone-refractory prostate cancer.

⌘ Biological markers for the detection and follow up of bladder cancer are being studied.